I CAN STILL DANCE THE MERENGUE !

A CELEBRATION OF WOMEN WITH BREAST CANCER

I CAN

STILL

DANCE THE MERENGUE !

A CELEBRATION OF WOMEN WITH BREAST CANCER

ALINE MENEZES
AND
DEREK JACKSON

Published by
Data Visuals, LLC
Foster City, California, USA
www.datavisuals.net

To Jennifer and Eric,
Here it is as promised.
Now where is your book Eric?
Not bad for a white kid eh?

Derek

(Thanks for your support.
Aline   08/19/03

I Can STILL Dance The Merengue!
Copyright © 2003 Aline Menezes, Derek M. Jackson, Data Visuals, LLC

Data Visuals, LLC
1125 East Hillsdale Blvd. Suite 112
Foster City, California 94404 USA

Telephone: 650 577-0990
Website: www.datavisuals.net

Printed and bound in the United States of America

ISBN 0-9742499-0-4

This book is divided into two basic sections. The first half deals in detail with Aline's battle – all her trials and tribulations, all the operations, each stage documented and photographed. She is the only topless woman here and she did that only to better show to those that follow her, what it all ends up looking like. She went from lumpectomy to mastectomy to reconstruction – the culmination of that being when the nipple was placed and the areola tattoo done – yes, you heard right – the surgeon uses a tattoo technique to get the colors right; amazing, isn't it?

Then, in the second half, come the rest of the women: Filipina, Brazilian, African-American, Native American, Mexican and Caucasian American.

I thought that you might be interested in how the various shots in the book came into being and maybe you are asking yourself – why is she riding a horse dressed as Cleopatra, or indeed why is she surrounded by all those masks – so I will explain.

All of the women were offered the opportunity to be photographed when, where and doing whatever they wished. It would be their day and my idea in giving them free reign was to expose the spirit and energy behind their cancer, to show them all STILL doing whatever it was that they loved to do. So, you will see Diana, dressed up as Cleopatra practicing her operatic voice, in fact singing Aida, if I remember correctly, while galloping around on her Arabian stallion. Julieta's thing was wigs, lots of them, and her work with animals, as she is an excellent veterinarian. Patricia and her masks come from her love of the musical genre. "Phantom of the Opera" was hereby invoked. Other ladies wanted to show their reflection, their tranquillity and, in some cases, even their faith.

Using this formula all the shots are different – different photographic techniques and equipment, varying from just a raw camera and film to a full scale production employing smoke machines and big lighting. (The smoke machine was great fun and Aline, my "camera assistant" on all the shoots, will, one day, learn to operate it!…)

Although most of the ladies are married with children, all, with the exception of Bonnie, wished to be photographed alone. It seemed that, although their family support system was invaluable, this was their personal battle.

So, I hope you enjoy looking at the girls. They all were stars for a day in front of a camera, although I know that they are stars each and every day.

Derek

The printing of this limited first edition was made possible by

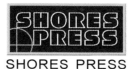

SHORES PRESS
1100 Industrial Road, Unit 2
San Carlos, CA 94070 USA
650 593 2802
www.shorespress.com

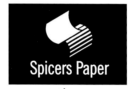

www.spicers.com

And by financial help from:

Julieta Gonzalez, DVM and Awesome Care
Lisa and Linda
James L. Adams, DDS, Inc.
Matthew C. Hudson and Pamela M. Hudson
The Ernle W. D. Young and Margaret M. Young Trust Agreement
Alliance of Chief Executives, LLC

••••••••••••••••••••••••••••••••••••

Part of the proceeds from the sale of this book will be donated to:
**The Community Breast Health Project, Palo Alto, California, USA
and Espaço Renascer at the Cancer Hospital, Recife, Brazil**

••••••••••••••••••••••••••••••••••••

Aline's dress for the back cover photo provided by Anett Schneider
www.anettcouture.com

"Your spirit is as beautiful as your physical presence...
The many women in this book have been brought together
to hopefully shed some positive light on cancer.
We are all in this together. Cancer does not always have to win...
We cannot let cancer take away our spirits."
(Brenda Paxton)

This limited first edition book can be purchased directly from the publisher:

Data Visuals, LLC
1125 East Hillsdale Blvd. Suite 112
Foster City, California 94404 USA
Telephone: 650 577-0990
E-mail: icanstilldance@datavisuals.net
Website: www.datavisuals.net

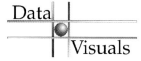

the ladies

Aline Lacerda de Menezes
Age 44 at diagnosis
Married
One daughter, 19
Small Business Owner/Homemaker
Foster City, California

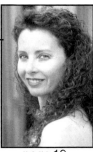

Antoinette Galindo
Age 44 at diagnosis
Married
No children
Real Estate Agent
Burlingame, California

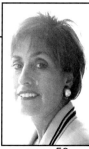

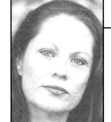

Liliane Lacerda de Menezes
Age 43 at diagnosis
Single
One son, 18
Travel Agent
Recife, Brazil

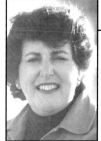

Patricia Jednorozec
Age 50 at diagnosis
Married
One son, 23
Dental Hygienist/Health Consultant
Palo Alto, California

Marianne Riddle
Age 42 at diagnosis
Married
Three sons, 20, 19, 13
Full time Mom
Burlingame, California

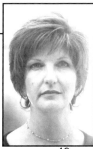

Diana Hoffman
Age 49 at diagnosis
Married
One son, 29
CEO of a California based company
Redwood City, California

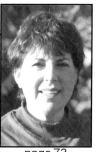

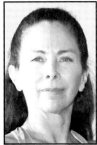

Terry Wyrsch
Age 40 at diagnosis
Married
One son, 21, one daughter, 19
Fitness Instructor
Foster City, California

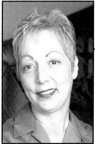

Nancy Petersen
Age 49 at diagnosis
Single
Two sons, 26, 18
Office Coordinator
Millbrae, California

Maria Santiago

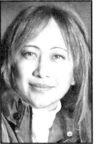

Age 33 at diagnosis
Married
One daughter, 9
Mail Carrier
San Francisco, California

page 85

Julieta Gonzalez

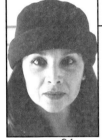

Age 43 at diagnosis
Single
No children
Veterinarian, runs her own clinic
Oklahoma City, Oklahoma

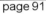
page 91

Pam Thunen

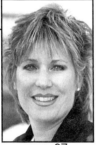

Age 37 and 42 at diagnosis
Married
Two sons, 24 and 19
Dental Assistant/Super-Mom
San Mateo, California

page 97

Maria José de Moura

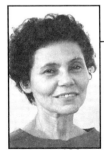

Age 44 at diagnosis
Single
No children
Retired
Recife, Brazil

page 103

Francicleide Torres Cabral

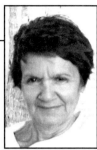

Age 38 at diagnosis
Married
Two daughters, 34, 32
Retired
Recife, Brazil

page 109

Aldira Roberta de Oliveira

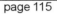

Age 34 at diagnosis
Married
One son, 21, one daughter, 18
Pharmacist
Recife, Brazil

page 115

Célia Muniz de Lyra

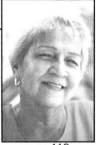

Age 58 at diagnosis
Married
No children
Retired Teacher
Olinda, Brazil

page 119

Bonnie Foster

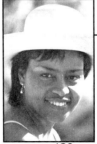

Age 33 at diagnosis
Married
One daughter, 15, one son, 6
Medical Salesperson
Edmond, Oklahoma

page 123

Brenda C. Paxton

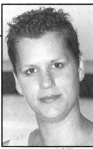

Age 33 at diagnosis
Married
One son, 10, two daughters, 13, 8
Business Owner/Mom/Student
Oklahoma City, Oklahoma

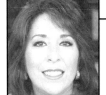

Cherokee Ballard

Age 35 at diagnosis
Single
No children
News Anchor/Reporter
Oklahoma City, Oklahoma

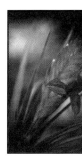

a few other things

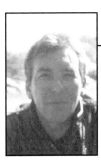

Letters from the Photographer

Group shots

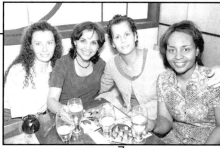

Bloopers

some of our best faces

Dictionary

What some of the
words we used mean.

biopsy
cancer
dcis
stage
tumor
x-ray

Resources

books
information
support
web sites

group shots

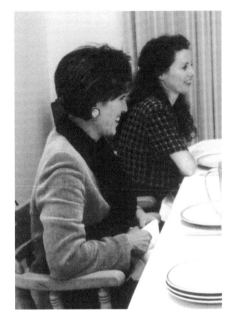

In California, Antoinette and Aline listen and amuse themselves...

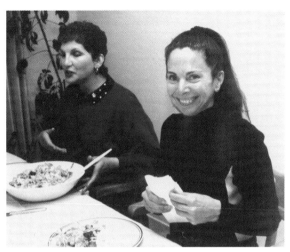

...as Marianne tells one of her silly stories. Terry seems entertained as well.

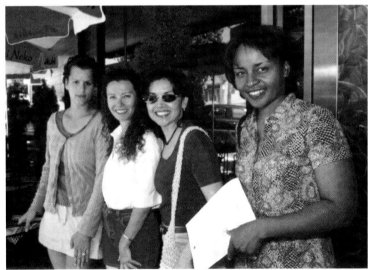

Aline with three of the Oklahoma City ladies: Brenda, Julieta and Bonnie.

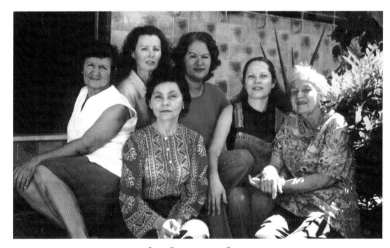

In Recife, the Brazilian women: Francicleide, Aline, Maria José, Roberta, Liliane, Célia.

introduction

from aline

Two weeks before a second partial mastectomy of my left breast I decided to be photographed because I was told that with the second surgery my breast would probably look very deformed. Although I have never been a vain person and have always disliked having my picture taken, I wanted to have the memory of what I looked like before the operation, especially because there was a good chance that I would have to have a partial mastectomy, if the new surgery didn't remove all the cancer.

I chose Derek to photograph me because he is a very perceptive man and because I love his work. I didn't want glamour shots, but I wanted the feeling of being affected by breast cancer and how I am to be captured in the photographs. I was never able to clearly explain to Derek just what I wanted, but he, being the artist that he is, took the most beautiful images that showed exactly what I had had in mind all along.

The photo shoot was fun, dramatic and emotionally charged. I went from happiness to sadness, from smiles to tears.

I absolutely loved the pictures, and so did everyone who saw them. They were not glamour shots, they were beautiful, artistic representations of me, who happened to be facing breast cancer.

At first I was determined that these photographs would remain my sole, very private property. However, after I arrived home from my surgery I kept thinking about something that Derek had said to me. He knows I love to dance, especially the Latin dances. After one of my several outbursts of sadness he looked at me and said. "Aline, it's like this: when you awake from your surgery tomorrow, you will still be able to dance the merengue. You will still be the person you are now."

So, as I rested in my recliner, I realized that I was about to put these poignant photographs in a drawer, where they would remain locked away. What a waste! I thought that there must be other women out there who would also like to be photographed and be part of an inspirational collection of pictures, and the idea of the book was born. I called Derek and we started working on this book right then and there.

from happiness to sadness

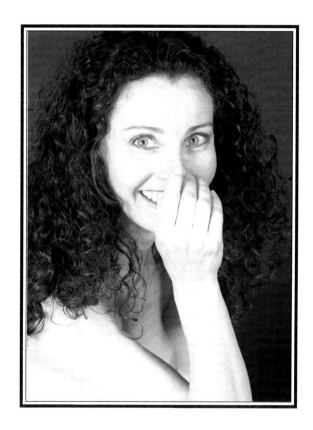

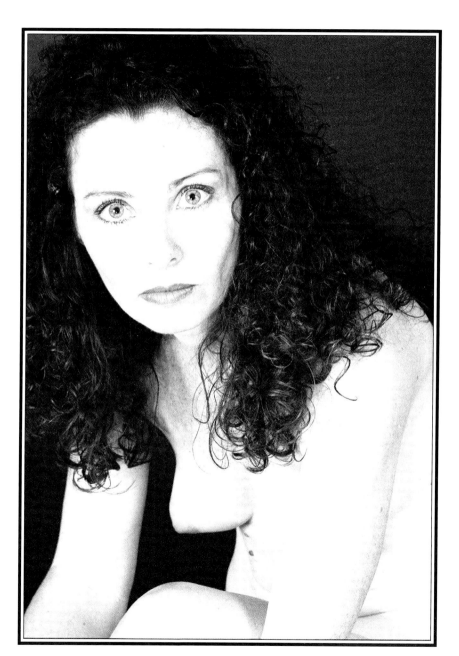

from smiles to tears

introduction

from derek

I worried as I took these photographs that I might be accused of "sanitizing" the issue. However, on reflection, they are not meant to be hard hitting medical shots. The object of this book is to portray these women, these rays of hope, these heroines, so that they might inspire and console others, that their lives, their families and the love they have would give a glimmer of light at the end of a dark tunnel. So, my shots are gentle, funny sometimes, thought provoking always, at least I hope that you, the reader, male or female, enjoy looking at them.

I hope my images and these ladies own words can help all of us affected by cancer or not, understand their pain and their joy and their determination. They have joined Aline to show to the world that they can STILL do the merengue, or aerobics, or deliver your mail or be the best moms in the world, just as before.

They are STILL the wonderful people they always were... They can STILL ...

My small part in this book is dedicated to my amazing friend Aline and indeed to women everywhere.

Derek M. Jackson
Photojournalist

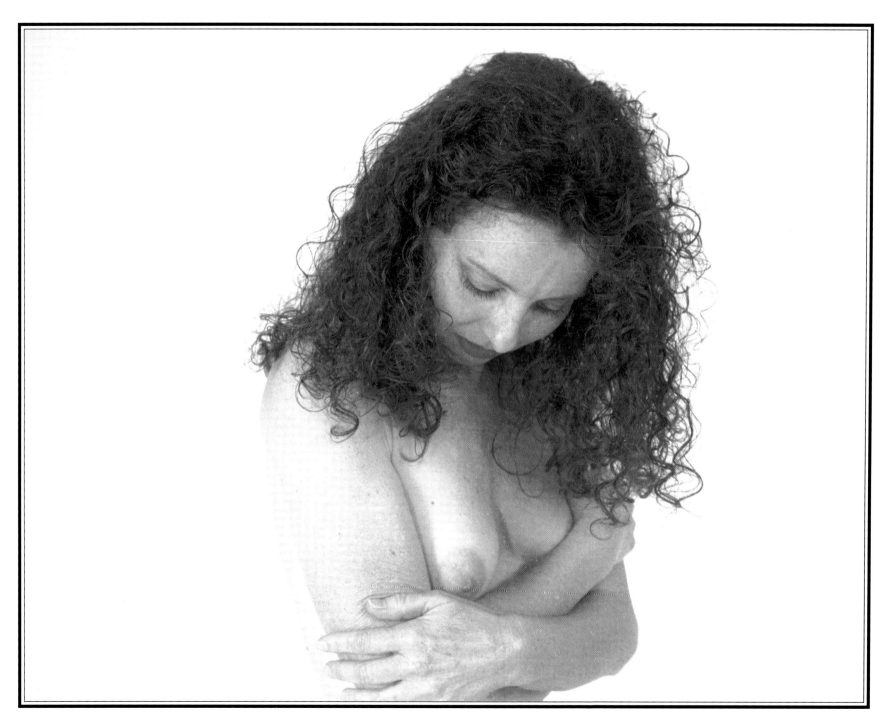

11

It was a sad day for those who loved Marianne and Nancy when they passed away after their long, long battles with cancer. We weren't quite finished with this book when they left us, but we decided to keep them as part of our celebration because, had we not, we wouldn't have been honest with ourselves, or with those they left behind or with the reality of life. It would have been as though we had denied their existence, their spirit, their legacy, the impact they had on our lives.
It was their wish to be included in the book.
We couldn't think of a better way to honor them.

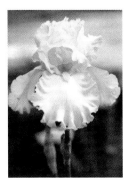

The reality today is that most of us diagnosed with breast cancer are able to beat it, and those who are unable to stay on this planet remain a part of our lives forever.
We hope that all the women in this book will inspire you and give you hope, courage and the strength to live your life one day at a time.
This book is for all of us who have been affected by cancer, one way or another.

To Marianne

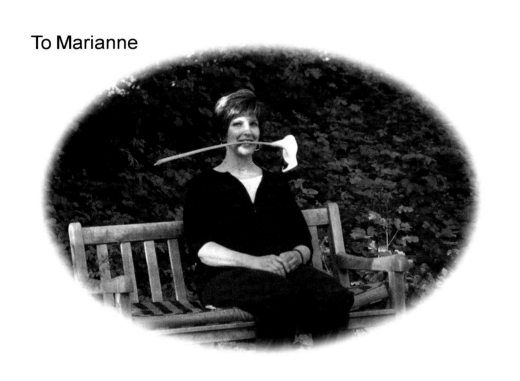

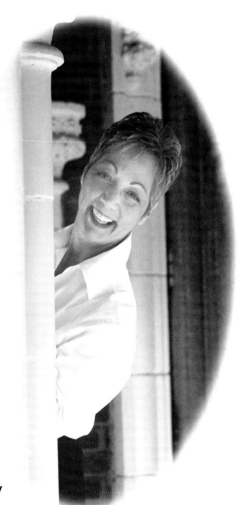

To Nancy

All of us in this book agree:
once you're faced with cancer and you feel that your life is in danger,
little things in life become exactly that...
little things.

....

I will be forever grateful
to those who walked my journey with me:

You listened, you laughed and you cried with me.
My husband and my girls, Sandra and Yeni. I love you.
My dear sister, Liliane and my brother, Sérgio. Amo vocês.
Manfred and Edith. Ich liebe euch.

Brian, Linda, Christina, Kate and Nancy.
Marie, for praying with me and for her wonderfully innocent, blunt questions and
comments (they put things in a simple perspective.)

Marianne Riddle.
Garret and Travis for holding Sandra's hand.

My dear friend and business partner, Derek, for being there, always, and for putting up
with my "occasional" moments of bossiness and obsessiveness
as we worked on this book   :-)

....

My radiologist and her staff for finding the tumor early enough
to make my cancer "curable".
My wonderful surgeon and Dr. Davis for taking such good care of me,
for their support and their endless patience.
The Community Breast Health Project in Palo Alto, California

"… I wanted my cancer to go away and leave me alone…
I didn't want to have to deal with it."

aline lacerda de menezes

my journey

December 14, 1999

I had the feeling my life was going to change today. My last mammogram had been a year or so ago. When the technician called me back for yet another film I knew that something was wrong. I wasn't afraid, thought that breast cancer was out of the question for me, but started looking at this brochure titled: "You've been told you have breast cancer". My radiologist told me that there were some micro-calcifications that hadn't been there in the previous mammogram. "We should check them out", she said.

A few days later

My gynecologist called and told me that I should probably have this new "finding" in my left breast checked. There was something there that the mammogram picked up, although neither the doctor or I could feel anything different in my breasts. She referred me to a surgeon, a breast specialist. I was beginning to worry that something might really be wrong. She thought I should have a biopsy done to make sure it was nothing.

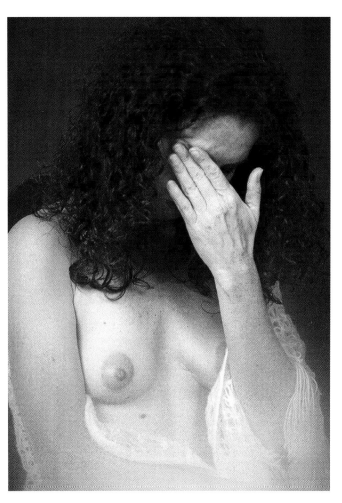

I was told I had breast cancer!

January 5, 2000

I saw a general surgeon who specializes in breast surgery, and she explained what she was going to do and why. I was scheduled for a biopsy on January 24.

January 24, 2000

It was a small growth according to the mammogram, and because it could not be felt by palpation or any other way, the radiologist inserted the wire inside the growth so the surgeon could find it and remove it. They call this a wire-localized biopsy. Then I headed for the hospital.

I had never been in a hospital before, except to give birth to my daughter sixteen years before or to visit someone. I had always been very healthy and did not want to accept this to be happening to me. I was nervous when I got to the hospital, and when I was about to be given the general anesthesia for the biopsy, I was scared that I would not wake up from the anesthesia or that something would go terribly wrong. I didn't want to die and leave my daughter without a mother. I remember crying with fear soon after the anesthesiologist gave me a sedative.

When I woke up I was told that everything had gone fine and that there had been no problems with the surgery. I went home the same day and to work the next.

A few days later
Waiting for the results of the biopsy was horrible. My surgeon told me that the pathology report said that the growth taken out were micro-calcifications: a 3 mm invasive tumor and a few areas of multifocal ductal carcinoma in situ (DCIS), and that the margins weren't clear around the sample taken.

I was told I had breast cancer!

I thought I was having a nightmare, I felt that my body had betrayed me, I had thoughts that I could die from this. My grandmother had died of breast cancer. I was only forty-four, I wasn't supposed to have cancer at this age! I had a family to take care of and there were so many things I wanted to do that I hadn't done yet.

I was devastated, but this was something that I didn't want to let defeat me. Although I hated the idea of being a victim to breast cancer I wanted to get rid of it and go on with my life as soon as possible, fight this head on and win.

Whenever I do something new that I know nothing about, or if I have some kind of project that is new to me, I like to first read a lot about it or learn as much as I can before I start working on it. I wanted to know what my options were and I wasn't going to decide anything without knowing what I was doing, or let anyone decide for me. I wanted to know exactly what was going to happen and how and why, every step of the way. The Community Breast Health Project in Palo Alto

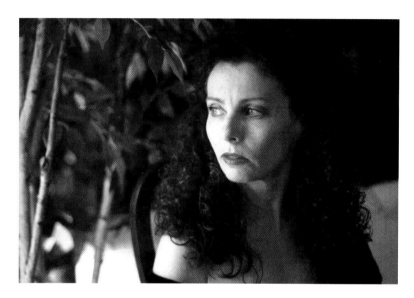

was a tremendous place for support and information for me. The women there, all somehow touched by breast cancer, welcomed me with open arms.

During the next ten days I had several tests done to look for any sign of spread: bone scan, liver function, chest x-ray, blood work ... There were no signs of metastasis or spread. I was thankful for that. At least the prognosis was good. Stage 1 breast cancer, the tumor was very small, no metastases, so I was scheduled for a lumpectomy and lymphnode dissection on February 14, Valentine's Day.

....

I felt generally good and happy, like I usually feel, most of the time. But I had moments when I thought I might go crazy, so, I cried a lot. Although I had so many other great things going on in my life, during those bad moments I felt alone, helpless, afraid and angry that I had this disease. I did not want to have to deal with this at this time in my life. My daughter avoided me and talking to me, but I knew that she was as frightened as I was. I wanted to give her time to deal with my disease, but, at the same time, I didn't want her to keep her feelings bottled up inside. I know how bad it is to keep your feelings to yourself.

I had always needed about eight hours of sleep, but now I started sleeping very little, tossed and turned a lot, kept waking up my husband with my restlessness, roamed around the house in the middle of the night. I found it difficult to go to sleep, and if I woke up in the middle of the night I couldn't make myself fall asleep again. I was having a really hard time dealing with the fact that I had breast cancer. This was not just a wound that, with time, would heal.

I talked about it with friends, with my husband, with my sister, who also had had breast cancer just a few years before. I found talking extremely helpful. Sandra and I also slowly started talking about it, but I got very upset every time I talked to her, because I knew that she too was upset about the whole thing.

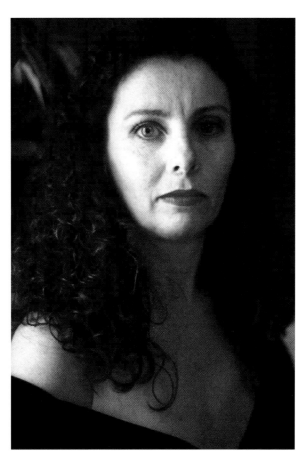

I know that my crying and my feeling so sad, depressed and helpless made her sad and upset. It was hard for all of us!

February 14, 2000
My surgeon was going to perform a partial mastectomy (lumpectomy) of my left breast and axillary dissection. There I was again, horrified with the idea of never waking up from the anesthesia and holding on to my husband's hand. He reassured me that everything was going to be fine.

In the recovery room, when I finally woke up, I remember asking the nurse if she was an angel and if this was heaven. She said: "No, I'm not an angel. I'm your nurse and you're in the recovery room. Everything went fine". I remember being very hungry and thirsty. When they moved me to my room, I asked for some food, but everything I tried felt very dry in my mouth and it was hard for me to swallow so I just had some soup, which was quite good.

I was hooked up to a morphine drip machine, which I didn't use much at all. I had expected to be in great pain, but I wasn't. I gave myself a shot of morphine a few times just so I would feel more comfortable. My husband stayed with me for a while and then he went home. I had a very restless sleep that night, I was sick to my stomach until they gave me something to stop the nausea. I kept waking up, watched some television (they show strange things at 3 a.m.) went back to sleep, and munched on my "delicious" dinner all night. I couldn't wait to go home.

In the morning, just before I was released, someone I didn't know stopped by to see me. It was a volunteer from a peer support program for women who have breast surgery at the hospital. She said she had come by to offer support, so we chatted for a little while. It was refreshing to see that there are strangers out there who will reach out and try to help someone and offer support. I appreciated her presence, her comfort and the few practical hints on, for example, what kinds of bras she found comfortable to wear after her lumpectomy.

I went home sometime in the morning. I was given a prescription for pain medication, but didn't really need it. I was surprised that I wasn't hurting more. I was told to take it easy, which is really hard for me because I like to be doing things all the time. If I am at home, I'm usually doing something, mostly housework, but also other things like gardening, fixing things perched up on top of a ladder, "playing" with my power tools. I'm a real man around the house!

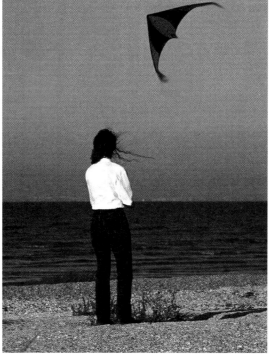

I can STILL fly my kite!

A few days later

Again, waiting for the pathology report was a real challenge. My surgeon told me that there was good news and bad news. I couldn't imagine what the bad news was. She told me the good news: the lymphnodes, twenty-three altogether, were clean, no sign of spread. The bad news: the margins were not clear and there are several multifocal DCIS.

I still had breast cancer! My world crumbled, and it seemed as if time stopped for a few seconds while I tried to understand what she was telling me. It was not supposed to happen like this. I was supposed to be free of cancer now.

A few days after the lumpectomy, my underarm started swelling and hurting so much that I could hardly move it. I knew there was fluid accumulated in there, but I didn't know it was going to hurt that much. My surgeon told me that indeed there was some fluid accumulated in my underarm area, but she assured me that it would soon be resorbed by my body. Within a few days I slowly and steadily was able to move my arm just as before the surgery.

I followed doctor's orders to stay at home for a week, and went back to work, as promised, a week, not a day later, after my lumpectomy. Thank God for work!

February 21 – April 6, 2000

The next several weeks were the most stressful weeks in my entire life. Most of the time I was emotionally fine because I kept busy at home and at work, I continued dancing as much as I could, but my disease was always in the back of my mind, and if I wasn't busy doing something I would be thinking about my cancer and what to do about it. During my bad moments I often became very depressed: I slept poorly, had little or no appetite, had a really hard time concentrating sometimes.

I thought, and so did everyone close to me, that I was dealing well with the whole thing. My life didn't really change much, the day-to-day was just like it had been before: work, family, home, dancing, friends, but the few moments in between day-to-day things were very tough.

During this period I saw three oncologists, one radiation oncologist, two plastic surgeons, two breast surgeons and one medical geneticist because I was considering genetic testing (there were three other women in my family who had had breast cancer). I also had an MRI of both breasts. All of the doctors except one of the oncologists and one of the breast surgeons, who said I might try a re-excision, recommended a mastectomy. I was extremely unhappy with the idea of losing my breast, especially because the cancer hadn't spread anywhere and because the tumors were fairly small. I also happened to really like my breasts and how they fit my body so well. I don't know

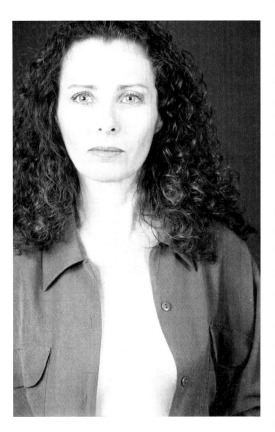

how many hours of my days and how many nights I agonized with the thoughts of one surgery versus the other: re-excision or mastectomy, and the impact that either one would have in my life, well-being and body. I talked with a few women from the Community Breast Health Project. I talked with my sister, my brother, my close friends, my husband and my daughter about my dilemma so many times. They were all wonderful and very supportive, and talking helped me put my thoughts together and just plain helped me get my fears off my chest. I cried so many times with them and in front of them. I don't know what I would have done without them. I cried almost every time I talked with my close friends and family about the decision now facing me. I had all these wonderful people around me and with me, but I felt so incredibly alone and lonely. None of them could really help me and make the cancer go away. No one could make it just disappear either, and that was what I wanted. I wanted it to go away and leave me alone; I didn't want to have to deal with it.

One day I went back to the Community Breast Health Project and the woman who greeted me asked me, after I had told her my dilemma, if I had looked at any pictures of women who had had breast surgery yet. I hadn't, of course, I didn't want to see what I would look like if I had a mastectomy. She told me that they had a book in the library, showed me where it was and told me I could come back and look at it whenever I was ready to do that.

I paced around the library for a while and decided to take a peak at the book. That was exactly what I did: I opened the book just enough to barely see the photos, just like you do when you're watching a scary movie and you look through your fingers in front of your eyes so you can't see the complete picture. When I finally got the courage to really open the book I saw photos of women who had had lumpectomies, and some of the breasts looked just like mine. As I turned the pages I also saw photos of women who had had mastectomies, both of one breast or bilateral, with reconstruction and without.

I was so glad I looked at that book! I found that the way some of the women looked after a mastectomy was acceptable, but somewhat deforming. Looking at those pictures made me decide that I should give myself another chance

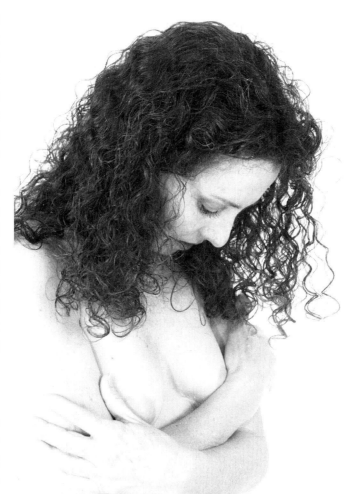

and just try a re-excision that might remove all cancer without having to completely lose my breast. It seemed like a reasonable decision.

When I saw my surgeon I told her that I really wanted to try and solve the problem with a second lumpectomy. She wasn't too happy about my decision, but agreed to do a re-excision. I really liked my surgeon for supporting me in my decision. She knew how difficult it had been for me to come to this decision.

After looking at the book at the Community Breast Health Project I thought it would be good to have my photos taken before the re-excision so I would have the memory of what my breasts and I looked like before the surgery. One day when I was talking to Derek, who had become one of my best friends, I told him about my idea and he immediately said he would love to take the photos. I got very excited about it because he is a great photographer, an artist really, very good at capturing feelings in his photos. So I had my photos taken and they were so amazing! Those first few photos are on pages 9, 11, 19, 23 and 24. Today I am so glad I did that.

April 24, 2000

I had my second lumpectomy, went home on the same day and waited, one more time, for the pathology report. I was told to once again stay home for a week to recover. Later that day at home after the surgery I kept thinking about my photo shoot - I must never be left alone with nothing to do but think "wonderful thoughts"- and I had the idea of creating a book about women who, like me, had breast cancer. The book would tell the world (and myself) that, for most women, there is life after you are diagnosed with breast cancer. When I first started thinking about the book I was trying to find the light at the end of the dark tunnel I felt I was in. There were actually a few reasons why I wanted to do this book. I thought it would help me heal emotionally and give me something really nice to work on. I wanted people to look at women with breast cancer and get inspired by their strength and their lives and by who they are, and see that there is so much more to them than their cancer. I wanted to

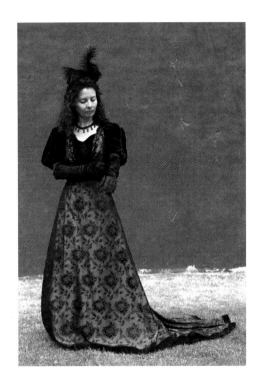

In western attire in Guthrie, Oklahoma, ready to join in the show with the Guthrie Gunfighters.

work with Derek on a project, and this seemed like it would be a good one.

So, here I was at home, waiting for the pathology report. Now, if waiting for the other two previous reports was difficult, waiting for this one was nothing less than painful. I really hoped, and so did my surgeon and everyone around me that it would be a good, clean report and that the next step for me would be radiation and tamoxifen.

A few days later

My surgeon told me that the news was not good: there was residual invasive ductal carcinoma, 7 mm in size. Additionally there was multifocal low-grade carcinoma in situ throughout. The margins were not clear. I still had breast cancer!

I wasn't upset when she first told me. My husband was out of town and I didn't have the courage to tell him the news over the phone when he called; I was numb. It hit me later on that I still had breast cancer and that it seemed like I had exhausted my options. It seemed like my body had made the decision for me: I had to choose between risking my life and losing my breast at this point. I was so unhappy for the next few days. I was so depressed, so anxious, so angry that I had lost this battle – but not yet the war.

When I saw the surgeon at her office on May 2, she told me how sorry she was for not being wrong. I knew what needed to be done next. We scheduled the total mastectomy for May 15. I also saw my plastic surgeon, Dr. Davis, that day, and we talked about the scheduled surgery. I wanted to start reconstruction immediately.

May 15, 2000

I was feeling extremely anxious that day. I disliked this breast cancer thing so much, but I knew that this is what I had to do now. At the hospital, after I talked to my surgeon, Dr. Davis came by and drew all over my breasts in preparation for his part of the surgery. I remember asking him if he was going to sign his artwork for me. As part of what had become some kind of routine, I began crying as soon as the anesthesiologist gave me the sedative. I have no idea how long the surgery lasted, but I'm guessing about three hours. After I woke up in the recovery room they took me to my room where my husband was waiting for me. I was so happy to see him! He helped me eat dinner and went home a little later.

Once again, I wasn't in a lot of pain at all, but my trusty morphine drip was hooked up to me, just in case. I just felt tired and hungry. My daughter Sandra, Travis and their good friend, Garret came by to visit me. They sat around and chatted for an hour or so and then left. I was so very happy to see them! I actually got to sleep that night, had a good breakfast and around mid-morning yet another lady from the peer support program came by to chat, see if I needed anything and offer support.

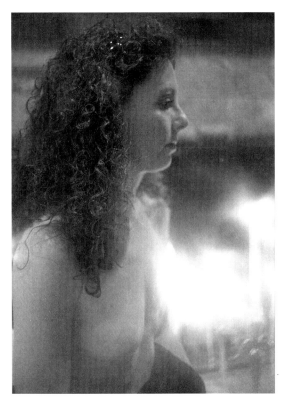

I chose to start reconstruction immediately. This photo shows the outline of the tissue expander.

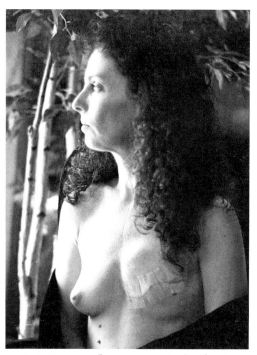

I got enough courage to look at myself in the mirror only several days after the mastectomy

A few days later

My surgeon called and left the message I had been waiting for. The pathology report looked good. The next step would be to see the two oncologists who had been following me and the radiation oncologist, get their opinions on what to do for treatment and start as soon as possible. Thankfully, I would not need radiation. Radiation could have make reconstruction difficult because of possible changes in the skin. I was told to stay at home for at least a week, not to lift anything heavy (that included pots and pans and laundry baskets (I really liked

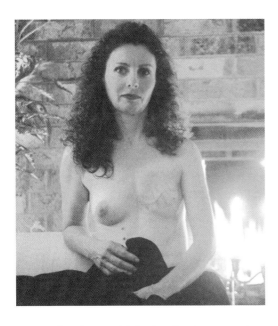

When we had scheduled the mastectomy and I was told that I was going to have to stay home for at least a week after the surgery, I called Derek and asked him to come to San Francisco then to photograph the first two of the ladies who would be in this book: my friends, Marianne (page 49) and Terry (page 55). He arrived just a few days after the surgery and we started running errands related to the photo shoots immediately. It was a nice, busy, productive weekend, and Derek got to lift and move the heavy things all by himself! The photos, as I had expected, turned out so beautiful!

I went back to work on Tuesday, a week after my mastectomy. Finding something to wear that didn't show the breast binder too much was a bit of a challenge and just a minor inconvenience.

May 22 – August 8, 2000
My surgeon called and told me about the pathology report: everything was fine! There were no other tumors, all the

that part), to wear the breast binder for two weeks, and not to drive or make sudden moves with my left arm. I followed Dr. Davis' orders, but it was really hard for me to take it easy because I felt so fine physically.

I felt a sense of relief now because I knew that the cancer was finally gone. I wasn't in great discomfort, but I did not like the way I looked. I took a look at what I was calling the "construction site" only several days after the surgery. I couldn't make myself look at it right away because I was afraid of my own reaction. Many days passed before I let anyone look at my chest.

Dr. Davis started filling the tissue expander in the beginning of June, when he was satisfied with the way the incision was healing.

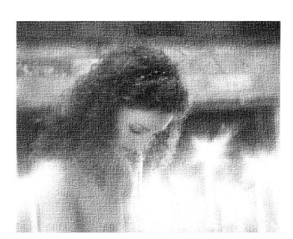

margins were clear, and so the prognosis was good. I was, of course, very, very happy to hear such good news!

I saw my two oncologists and the radiation oncologist to discuss any other treatment. They were all of the opinion that I didn't need radiation or chemotherapy, and all they were recommending was tamoxifen for five years, with a trial period of a few months to see how well I tolerated the medication. That was such excellent news!

Over a period of several months, I went to Dr. Davis's office six to eight times to fill the tissue expander and when it was fully expanded, I looked like I had half a grapefruit stuck under my skin where my left breast used to be. I had to keep reminding myself that this was only temporary and that in a few months it would be replaced with the final implant that would match my other breast. It was almost twice as large: it was over expanded to make enough room for the final implant, so that when it was put in, the implanted breast would appear naturally droopy like the other breast.

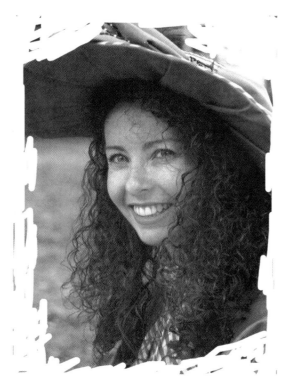

I know I was very lucky in the sense that the cancer was caught very early on and that,

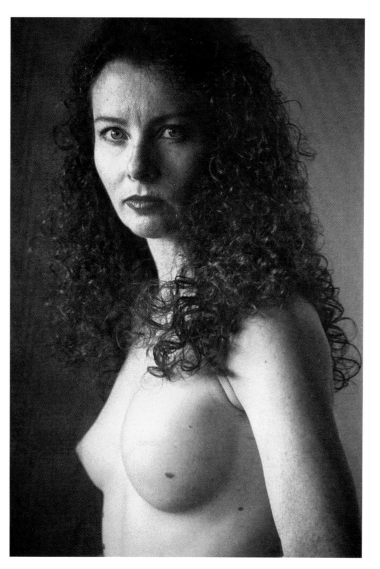

The tissue expander, filled to its fullest to make room for the implant in a few months. I used to call it my "grapefruit".

28

according to the way things were going, it looked like I was probably going to be fine for many years. I was very aware of the fact that things could have been much worse. I was thankful that it was fairly easy to treat my cancer and that there was no sign of spread, and that, for the time being, I was free of cancer.

August 26, 2000
In the few weeks that followed I saw myself once again doing things that I used to do before the diagnosis and that I had not done in a while. I had put so many things on hold and also neglected so many things, such as my plants that I always took such good care of. I had a red hibiscus outside and I nearly killed it by neglecting it and I had had it for almost nine years. I took a good look at it one day and realized that it was in desperate need of some care. It felt great to go back to taking good care of my plants again.

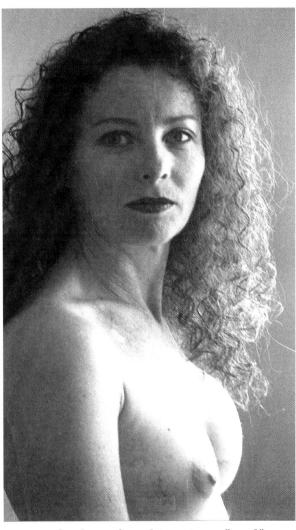

A few days after a biopsy in my "good" right breast.

I went shopping one day because we needed to get a few things and when I came back I went on a cooking spree. That was how it used to be before. When I got home and started cooking, once again I had this feeling of the haze dissipating, a deja vu feeling. It was like one of Marianne's photographs, the one on page 50 with the smoke all around her, but then it felt like it was slowly disappearing, bit by bit as the weeks went by. It was a good feeling!

September, 2000
The tissue expander was full to a reasonable size, and we were just waiting for the muscle and skin to settle so the permanent implant could be put in. For a while I was undecided on what to do about my right breast. I had the option to leave it alone, but then it would be a different shape than the left one, or to enlarge it a little bit so that it would match the left side better. As far as I knew matching sizes in breast reconstruction is fairly easy, but matching the shape of the other breast requires some kind of surgery. An implant on the right side could make monitoring the right breast a little more difficult.

September 28, 2000
I saw my surgeon today for my four-month follow up after my mastectomy. Everything looked fine, the scar was healing well, and she was happy with the way the

Now, when I did something that I had not done for a while, it was as if a haze was being lifted and I could see more clearly.

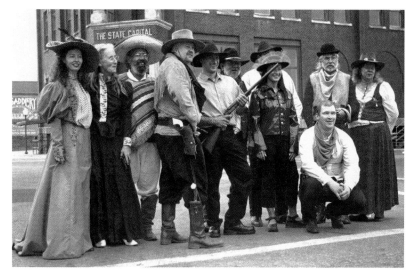

I can STILL dress up and spend fun days with the Guthrie Gunfighters in Oklahoma

expander looked. As she examined what I thought was my "good" right breast I saw her face change. She felt a pea size lump that didn't seem to have been there before. I was not happy to hear that and I was afraid that this would be the beginning of yet another journey. She wanted an ultrasound to get a better idea of what it might be.

October 4, 2000
I went to the radiologist's office for an ultrasound of my right breast and, right after that, to my surgeon's. There was definitely a growth there, some blood vessels around it were making it hard to determine what it could be. I immediately agreed with the suggestion of having it looked at, so we scheduled a biopsy for October 9. Here we go again... I didn't tell a lot of people about this new finding because I wanted to know what it was first. I was, of course, very worried about it, and kept thinking about what to do if it was another tumor. I put off any decision about the reconstruction until this new issue was resolved.

October 9, 2000
So there I was again. I already knew the routine after being at this hospital four times. I recognized some of the staff there and that actually amused me. Life can be so "interesting"!

Everything seemed to have gone very smoothly. Once again I had to wait for the pathology report. The few people who knew about it and I were anxiously waiting to hopefully receive good news. Waiting was no easy task for any of us!

A few days later
Good news, very good news! The report said that no carcinoma or intraductal carcinoma was present. The biopsy showed proliferative fibrocystic change with a large dilated cyst. I could live with that. I was so happy and relieved to hear the good news. I celebrated later in the evening with a bottle of champagne. All photos showing the tissue expander at its fullest (I affectionately called it the "grapefruit") were 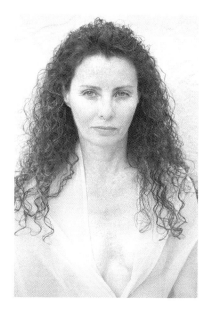 taken about a week after the biopsy in my right breast.

30

October 2000 - January 2001

As I waited for the tissue and muscle to settle I kept thinking about what to do about the implant. As I mentioned before,

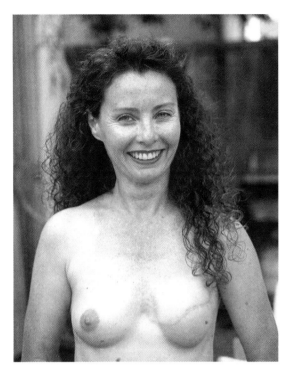

I was happy with the way my new left breast matched the right one.

for a while I considered augmenting the right side for two reasons: to better match the left side in shape and size and to just have slightly bigger breasts. But why did I need bigger breasts? I liked them the way they had always been. In the end I chose to leave the right breast alone because augmenting my good breast would make it more difficult to monitor it, and

since I already had a scare and a strong family history of breast cancer, I thought it would be wise to leave it alone and not try to fix what was not broken.

January 25, 2001

I thought it was somewhat ironic that my reconstruction surgery was scheduled for a day exactly one year after the first biopsy. I saw it as a good sign.

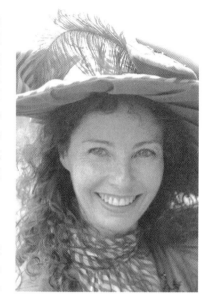

My husband and my daughter both went to the hospital with me and stayed around until I was taken to the operating room. Once again I cried as I said good-bye to them when I was wheeled away to the operating room - I was always worried that something might go wrong. I remember asking Sandra to tell Marianne that I loved her.

I was told that everything went as planned and I was able to go home the same day. The grapefruit was gone and was replaced by what I then called a half orange that matched the size of my right breast really well. After the bandages came off and I looked at myself I was very happy with the results, the way that I fit in my clothes again and that I didn't look lopsided anymore.

May 15, 2001

Once again it was somewhat ironic that I had an appointment with my surgeon on this day that I will remember forever: exactly a year ago today she performed a mastectomy of my left breast. I was a little anxious going back to see her, but I think I will be anxious every time I have a routine appointment, as I watch the doctors examine me, as I wait for them to tell me that everything looks fine. It was a good appointment, a happy anniversary: everything looked great according to her and I was extremely glad to hear that.

July 20, 2001
The last step, hopefully the final chapter in my cancer journey: the tattooing of the areola and nipple reconstruction. I was very happy with how I looked after the stitches were removed and I could look at myself in the mirror and see that my new breast now seemed complete. All my other doctors agreed that Dr. Davis had done a really good job and that my skin healed very nicely.

Today I feel blessed, lucky and thankful for being alive and doing so well.

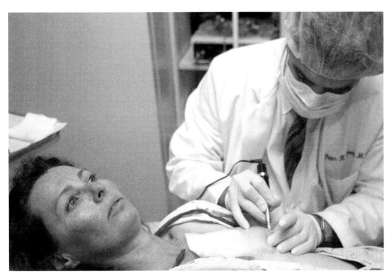

Dr. Davis tattooing my new nipple.

I would like to say to anyone who is trying to make a decision about breast cancer treatment that there are other options that I have not mentioned here. The decisions I made for my treatment were those that worked best for me and you should not assume that I am recomending them to you. All the women in this book and many other women I talked to all had different experiences and made very diverse choices as they fought breast cancer. What you choose for yourself should be based on your own situation and issues. I wish you only the best.

September, 2001: My final thoughts
As we approach the end of putting this book together I often reflect and think about the past eighteen months. It has been a long journey, a roller coaster ride that has forever changed the way I look at life. Having cancer has made me realize how very fragile we really are, and that, therefore, we must live each moment to its fullest. I don't let little things bother me anymore and I try to treasure the good, important things because they are really what matter. I make sure to let those who I love know that I love them and that I am there for them if they need me. I was never a person to care much for material things and that feeling has become even stronger.

As I battled breast cancer, my life continued pretty much as normal as ever. Wait, actually, it didn't. In between surgeries and amidst many, many emotional ups and downs, I danced, I laughed, I cried; I worked, I cooked, I did the dishes and the laundry; I quit my job and started my own small business; I went to the movies, to dinners with friends and to my daughter's games and graduation; I rode roller coasters, watched a soccer game from the sidelines and spent carnaval with my family in Recife, Brazil. I pretended I knew

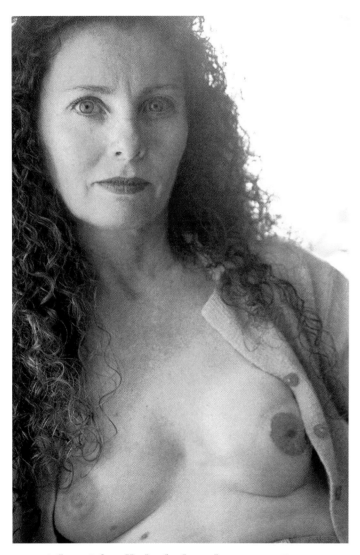

*When I finally looked in the mirror I saw
that my new breast seemed complete.*

what I was doing when I became "photographer's assistant" as we photographed the women for this book. When I visited my friends in Oklahoma City I watched drag-racing at Thunder Valley; I learned to target shoot pistols and rifles, I rode on the back of my friends' motorcycles. I visited a Navajo Indian Reservation in Arizona.

I made three of my dreams come true: I bought a stunt kite and learned to fly it, I went to the Amazon River Basin and I flew over the Grand Canyon. For a lot of us who have cancer, life does go on one way or another. Cancer has taught me to truly appreciate life.

....

May, 2003

A long time has passed since we first started working on this book and we are finally going to press! As I try to make the deadline the printer gave me to make all the necessary changes in the book, I realize that this is my last chance to say something that will hopefully comfort someone who has been diagnosed with a disease, of any kind really.

It is hard to hear the doctors say you have cancer. It is hard for those who love you to see you cry when you are told the news, but it is okay for all of us to cry and have strong feelings, good or bad. I think it is important to let your family and friends hold your hand and walk with you as you go on your journey.

As I battled breast cancer I made three of
my dreams come true

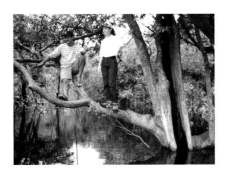

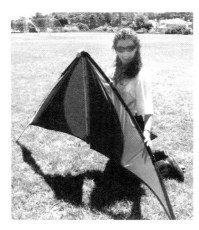

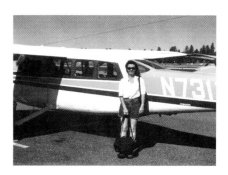

I bought a stunt-kite and
learned to fly it...

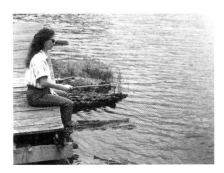

I went to the Amazon Basin...

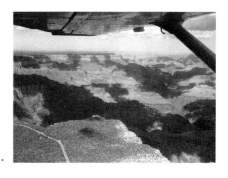

I flew over the Grand Canyon...

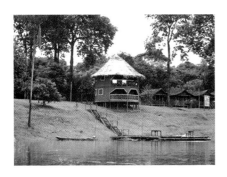

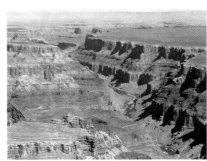

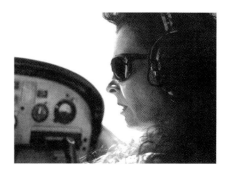

I also

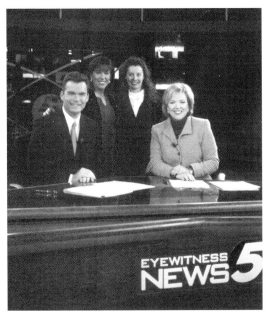

saw tv
from the inside

played gunfighter
in Guthrie

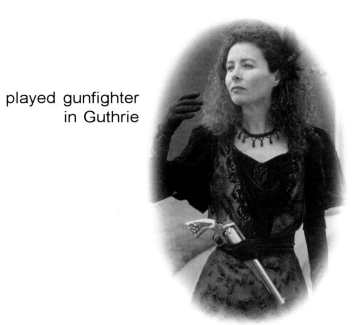

experienced the
passion of
Brazilian
soccer
from the pitch!

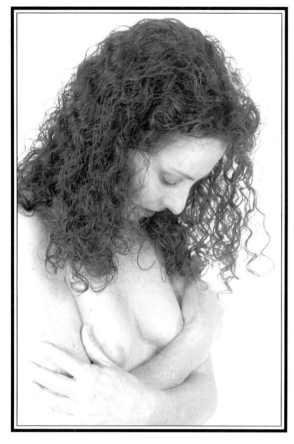

April 2000, just days before the
second lumpectomy.

before, during, after

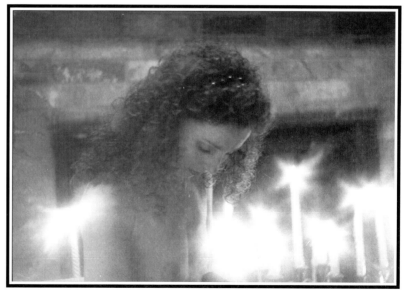

May 2000, two weeks after the mastectomy.

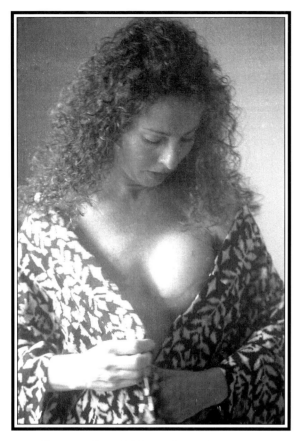

September 2000, when the tissue expander was at its fullest stage to make room for the final implant.

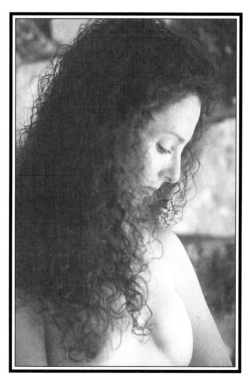

January 2001, a few weeks after the implant was put in.

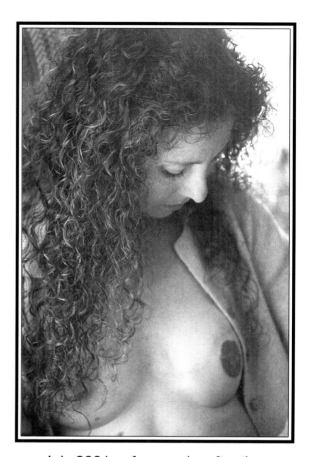

July 2001, a few weeks after the nipple reconstruction and tattooing of the areola.

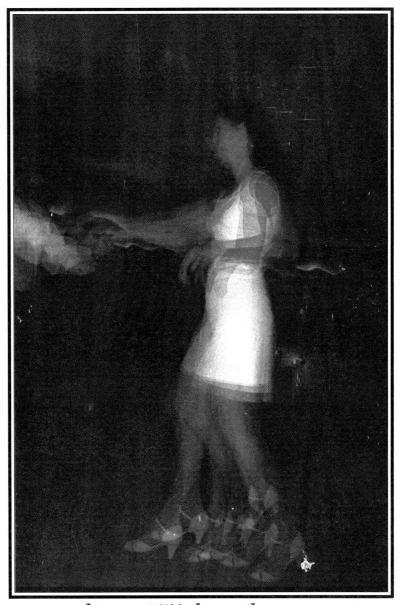

... and I can STILL dance the merengue!

Letter from the photographer

It was just past midnight in Oklahoma City when the phone rang. I was just finishing off my glass of scotch. "Aline in San Francisco here. Derek, I have a sort of special request". Aline went on to elaborate about her cancer and her desire to be photographed before her surgery. I readily agreed to take on the assignment, although I tried to make it clear to her that I was not a glamour photographer and that my point of view would more than likely be more documentary than pretty.

Aline arrived and the very next morning the shoot was arranged. It was to be an emotional moment. Aline laughed, then sobbed, she begged me to stop firing the shutter. I took no notice and kept on working. I knew we had some of the best photographs I had ever taken long before the film was processed. (Six photos from that shoot that we selected for this book are on the cover and on pages 9, 11, 19, 23 and 24). In fact, those shots were on the first roll of film. It was over; Aline flew home with her photos, a very private moment in time for her, the shots destined to become memories locked away in a drawer.

She returned from her surgery with what seemed like a new-found mission. I received another call... "Derek, it's a waste, isn't it? To keep these photos hidden... They could be inspirational to other women, couldn't they? Why don't we do a book? I jumped up with a start. "That's it, Aline, that's what we just have to do!"

Derek Jackson
Photojournalist

aline and liliane

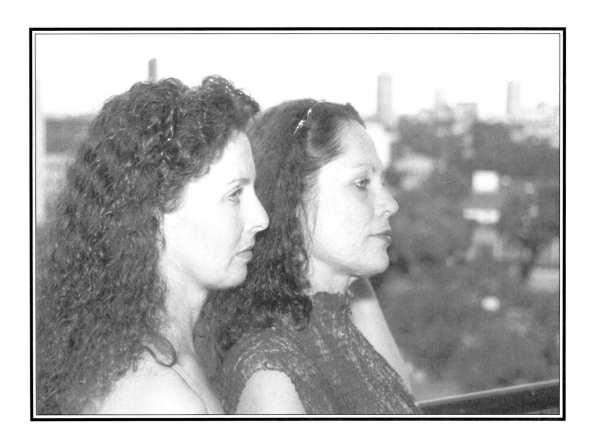

sisters…

liliane and aline

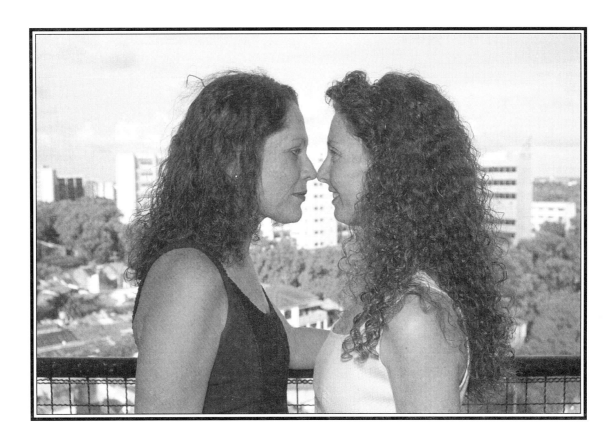

... sisters

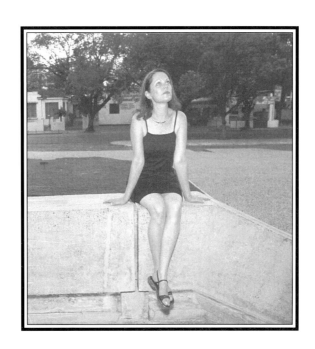

"For me the best medicine was to realize that the sun
continued to shine, that the sky was still full of stars…"

liliane lacerda de menezes

I can STILL love!

The first time I had cancer I was only thirty-three. They took my uterus and one of my ovaries. I was in shock in the beginning and all I could think about was my toddler son and what would happen to him if I died. My worrying about his future was much larger than the issues with the cancer itself, which, I must confess, were not hard to overcome. After the cancer was removed my life slowly got back to its normal routine.

Many years later, in 1998, when I found out that I had breast cancer I was devastated. I had my son, then twelve, and a quadriplegic aunt to take care of and who needed me to keep my wits. Today, I am certain that they were the best treatment and medicine for me at the time. I just had to beat breast cancer. It didn't matter what I would have to go through, I just needed to survive so I could continue providing for them.

There were some very bad moments when I felt very alone, being single and not having someone to share my fears with. The lumpectomy, the chemotherapy, the loneliness, the fear of the unknown and mainly the fear of maybe losing the battle were difficult, to say the least. My father

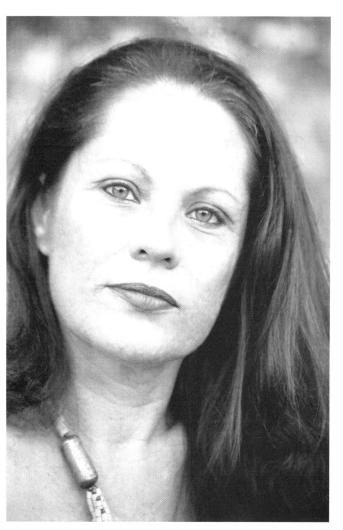

had died of stomach cancer just a few months before I was diagnosed with breast cancer. I thought about him constantly because he lived only two and a half months after his cancer was discovered. We lived in the same house for many, many years, so I was with him every day and every night throughout his last few months of life. He died at home, in my arms. I imagined that the same could happen to me if I didn't beat cancer. It was of the utmost importance that I win. All I knew was that I had to get better for my aunt, for my son and for myself. I continued working as much as possible during my treatment.

My aunt, my dad's sister, raised my three siblings and me from the time I was seven years old, she took us into her home and became our mother. She had lost her speech ability with the stroke that made her quadriplegic and remained that way for nine years before she passed away. She had been a very strong, gentle kind of person. She knew me like no one else and was able to comfort me with her soft yet strong ways, even without being able to utter a word. She saw and understood what I was going through and often "spoke" to me with her eyes and told me to be strong, that I was going to make it. And I did.

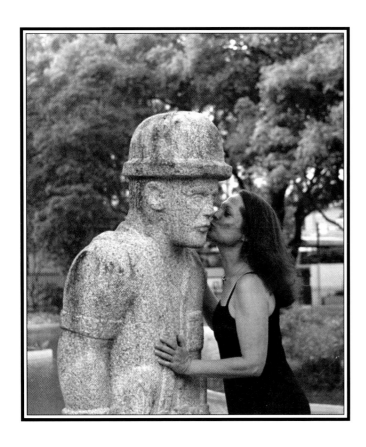

Today, I can still be silly...

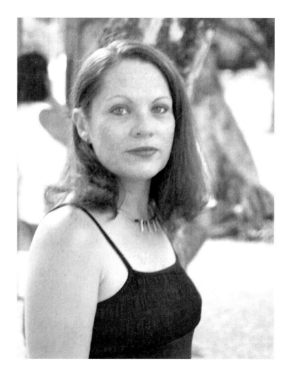

I found out during that time that my faith in God was what gave me hope, I discovered that you have to believe in something and fight for what you want. The secret for me was not to give in and not to think that I was less of a woman just because part of my breast had been taken away.

The best medicine was to realize that the sun continued to shine, that the sky was still full of stars, that the sea was still mysterious and beautiful, that the trees continued to flower and give fruit, in short, that life kept on going no matter what. I realized that the only thing the surgeon had taken from me was the cancer. What I was, knew, believed in and felt had remained part of me.

Now, 2002, I am still alive and happy. My aunt is now in a better place, my son is eighteen, and two of his friends have "adopted" me as their mother, so now I also have an adopted granddaughter.

It gives me great pleasure to share my cancer story with other women that have walked, are walking, or will walk the same path as I did. We are capable of fighting for our lives under the most stressful circumstances; we are all able to win, one way or another. It's not an easy battle, but it is possible to win it.

Today, I can still laugh, I can still be silly, I can still love, I can still work. I am still alive and I thank God for the second chance as often as possible! The essence of who I am remains untouched, more mature, yes, but untouched, and that's what really matters to me.

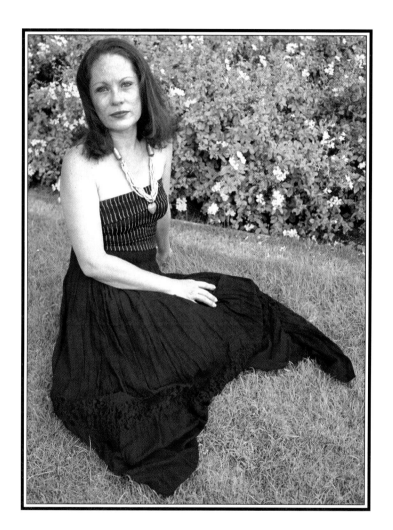

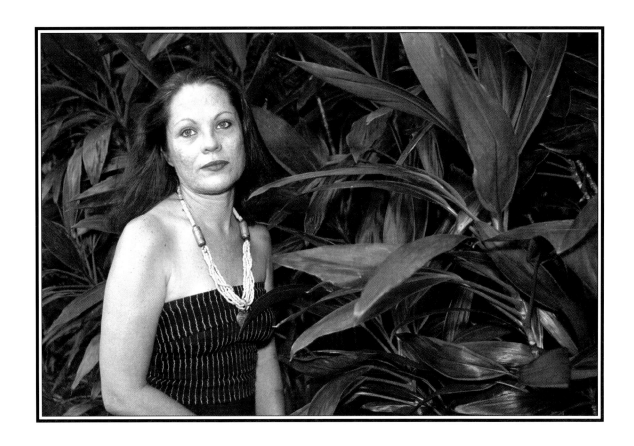

The essence of who I am remains untouched...

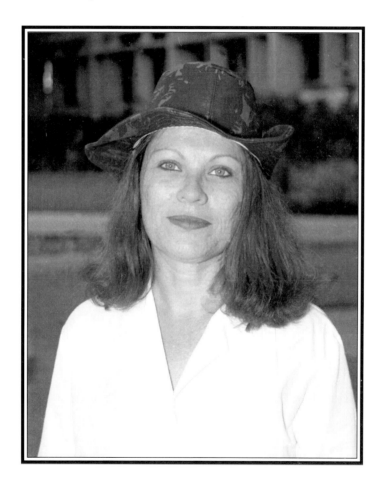

"... cancer does have its upside...
the sky is bluer, flowers are more vibrant,
the sun's warmth like a hug..."

marianne riddle

I can STILL laugh!

Laughter has always been a huge part of my life. I was raised in a wonderful family by loving parents who unburdened my life so I could fill it with laughter. I married a man with an incredible sense of humor who loved to make me laugh and we have raised our three boys to understand that a sense of humor can rescue them from almost any situation. Consequently, they understand humor and have taken my husband and me by surprise with a straight face and a simple sentence sending us into gales of belly laughs.

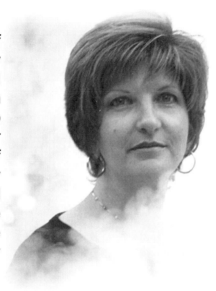

Humor also has rescued me from the fears of breast cancer and today, from cancer that has metastasized to my liver. I was diagnosed with breast cancer six years ago on February 26, 1995, and can vividly remember the drive home from the grocery store, feeling happy, as I sang a favorite old song on the radio. I don't know why that has stuck in my mind but I suppose it was because it was the end of my innocence. I hadn't been thinking about the needle biopsy on a lump found in my right breast when I took the phone call that changed my life. I wasn't frightened, just shocked, that I could have cancer. How was this going to affect my life? How would I tell my family? How would I tell my friends? Would I tell my friends? And, worst of all, how would I tell my parents?

I tested out the news on a girlfriend that I was seeing that afternoon. I told her the biopsy had come back positive and that I had breast cancer. I don't know what I was expecting, but her reaction surprised me. She jumped out of her seat, with quivering hands and tears in her eyes and hugged me fiercely, and only then did the severity of what was happening to me sink in.

I decided to share the news with everyone I cared about for two reasons. First, they were all important enough to me that I didn't want them to hear about it through the grapevine. I had many friends and acquaintances who shared parts of my life, and I felt it important to share this life-changing news with them. The second reason came to me as I tried to find meaning in the why me category, although I have never, to this day, asked that question in earnest. I decided if my story could convince one woman to get a mammogram who might otherwise have put it off or could be a resource to a newly diagnosed woman, then being wide open with the news would be worth it. The decision to give part of myself to others came back in more ways than I can count.

I made it through seven months of chemotherapy by keeping

my sense of humor as I hit highs (when I was off chemo) and lows - a few too many to count - but still seeing the end of the road as I pictured Thanksgiving dinner (which would mark the end of chemo) and a toast to life. I almost staged the toast to replicate what I kept in my mind at every chemo IV, Thanksgiving dinner, and that day was one of the happiest in my life.

The next nine months were interesting. I wasn't on a high as I started my life post- breast cancer. The chemotherapy took me from being premenopausal to postmenopausal in one month. I had symptoms of menopause through the chemo but was too wrapped up in trying to stay as normal as possible for my family to let it bother me. Now it was taking its toll. The hot flashes were manageable because they were obvious and boy, were they obvious! It was as though a little light would shine in the center of my body and radiate the heat outward with enough energy to light up a room. I dipped into the bag of holistic medicines to ease myself through almost everything, but there was still something I couldn't put my finger on and only after a visit to my primary doctor did he identify the depression... Depression? I took some sample antidepressants, but kept cutting them down to a smaller size because I didn't like the way they negated every emotion. I was down to the very last pill the day my father died suddenly and I threw the pill in the garbage.

His death brought my emotions back. I mourned the loss of his spirit from the depths of my soul and in doing so, found my own spirit again. I was able to put breast cancer in the past and live every day with the renewed joy of being alive to watch my children grow.

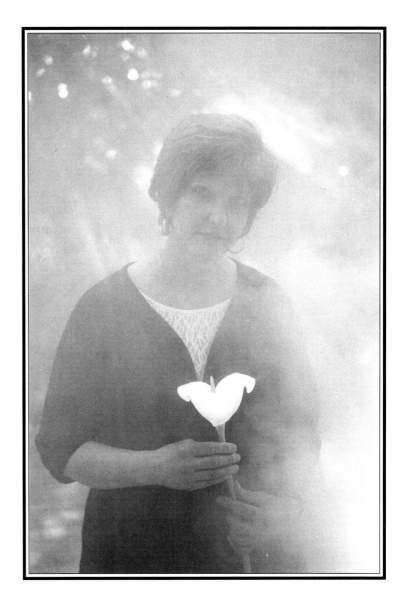

still be a mom....

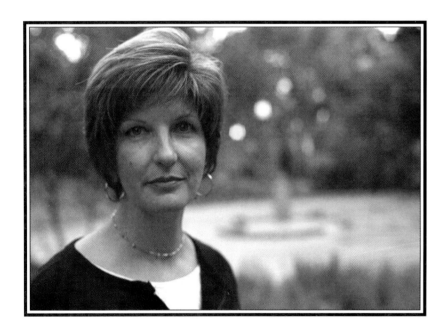

Cancer does have its upside. The sky is bluer, flowers more vibrant, the sun's warmth like a hug, laughter is joy and love is what life is all about. We slow down to appreciate EVERYTHING.

On June 20, 1999 I learned the cancer had returned and now I had to fight for my life. The news put me into a state of panic that became my constant companion 24 hours a day. Knowing I was going to die around my current age of forty seven instead of reaching an older age was unfathomable, the panic I felt was like losing track of a young child in a large crowd of strangers and gasping for breath in shear panic. That was the feeling I lived with until a biopsy could be done on my liver, the results known, and my oncologist telling me not to despair... There were lots of things we could do. It's now almost two years later and I'm doing remarkably well. I've been on three different types of chemotherapy, lost most of my hair, gained a bit too much weight, but through it all, I've kept my sense of humor.

The pictures of me were taken in a prayer garden by my home in Burlingame, California. The community of religious and spiritual people who own the land are loving and generous in opening their hearts and home to those of us in need. I attend a cancer support group there with people who come many miles to be in the presence of loving spiritual supporters. I chose the location for the deeper connection I've developed with God.

I love my family... I love my friends... I love my life.

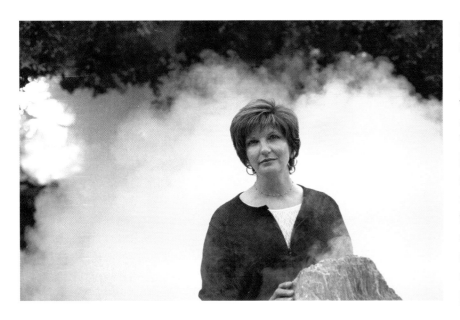

Epilogue to Marianne's Story

"When I run I can't cry..."

"To my beautiful family... I'll love you with the warmth of the sun. I'll kiss you in the gentle breeze of the afternoon. And I'll hug you tight as you lay sleeping." These were the words Marianne used to conclude her journal entry on July 16, 1999, one year, eleven months and one day before she passed away on June 17, 2001 from a disease that was first discovered in her breast, then her liver and finally her brain. She knew then what none of us were willing to believe or to accept until her final months, that her life with us would not be long. She left three sons, a husband, a mother, a sister, her dog, her cat and many, many friends and relatives. So now, those of us who so loved her are left to pick up the pieces - each of us, in our own way, trying to make sense of a life lost and a love now gone.

Marianne was many things to many people, but to me, she was my wife, my lover, my mentor, my soul-mate, the mother of our children, and my best friend for more than 20 years. We did everything together, our thoughts, actions, desires, beliefs and dreams so intertwined. So many experiences shared, and so much love given to one another. I clearly understand now how a marriage is indeed the joining of two individuals into one being, as the emotional support, counsel, companionship and love I have been so accustomed to, are no longer there for me. The better half of me is now gone and I am left to rediscover myself, my purpose and my being. I often hear that time heals; however, I've learned that time has nothing to do with healing, only a way to measure the distance from the passing of one I so adored, loved and now miss so deeply. Marianne found an "upside" to cancer, such a typical reaction of hers to adversity. She discovered a new purpose and determination for living. Her senses were enhanced and she saw the love and beauty of this world in ways not always seen or felt before. She opened her heart and mind to the realities of a spiritual self, and the peace and comfort that are there for us, even in great tragedy. How easy it would have been for her to quit, to give up on hope, to wallow in self pity, and to be to others what cancer was doing to her physically. How easy it would have been to remove herself from her family and friends, to give up on God and to let fear encompass her. But her courage and strength were boundless, and along the way she taught me what I needed to know to survive without her. How easy it would be for me to choose fear over courage, despair over hope, self pity over determination, and even death over life. However, Marianne's life was not about giving in or taking the easy way out, so, I look to her life as I try to find the strength and courage to continue mine in the solitude that her death brings.

Rarely a day goes by that I don't cry for the loss of her being. The pain is just too great not to, and so much of her physical life surrounds me. But I find that when I run, I can't cry. I find that when I run, my mind, body and spirit come together and I have a strong sense of a communion with her spirit. I'm not sure why I have such experiences, but I always find them comforting and her spirit has not disappointed. So I run often, and I run now with a purpose. Perhaps running is a good metaphor for dealing with the realities and pain of such a loss, to keep moving forward, one stride after another...

Brock C. Riddle

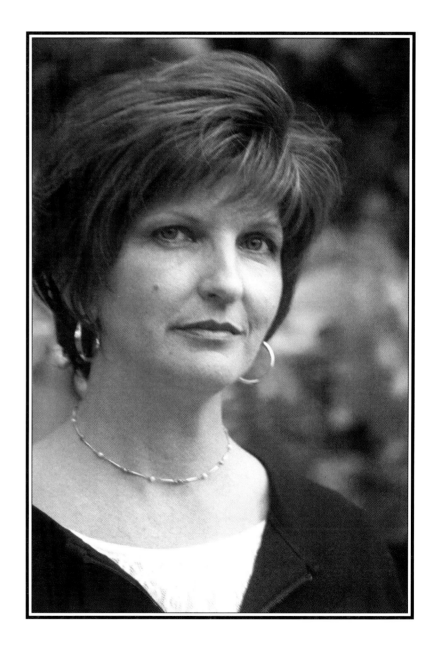

anyone
for
tennis?

terry wyrsch

I can STILL beat most men in tennis. I can STILL serve and they can't return my serves.

The Beginning:

My cancer was aggressive. I had a modified radical mastectomy (all breast tissue, some muscle and twenty three lymph nodes) in May 1993. Full reconstructive surgery followed in September of the same year.

I am in charge!

Not recovering was simply not an option. Nor was not being able to participate in the sports that I loved so much. This ordeal was going to be a temporary inconvenience – period! I planned on seeing my two great kids have children of their own. I planned on celebrating my fiftieth anniversary with my wonderful husband.

Temporary inconvenience:

A mastectomy is not as physically impairing as one might imagine. Two days after the surgery I attended my son's all-star baseball game. The next day my husband and I took a forty-minute walk and went out to dinner with eight friends. One week after the surgery I shot a video demonstrating a treadmill for a department store. Two weeks after the surgery I returned to teaching my fitness classes. I would say that at four and a half weeks I was

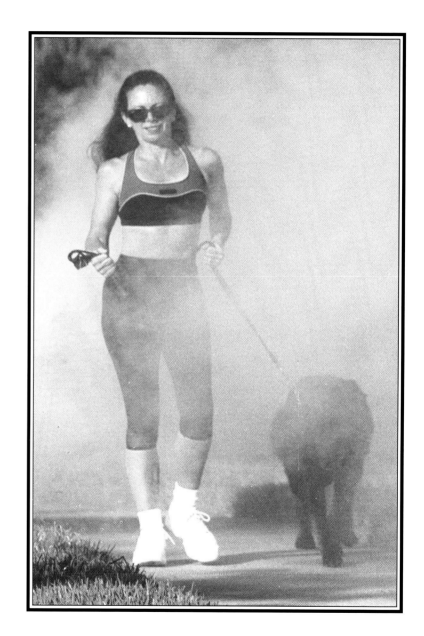

Remember: you will be able to do ANYTHING after breast surgery that you did before! There are no limits. You should, of course, consult with your doctors before starting any exercise program.

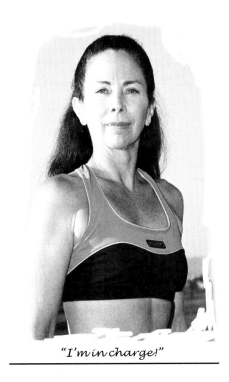

"I'm in charge!"

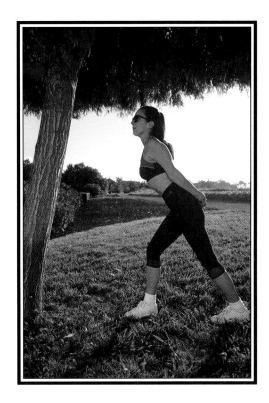

able to participate in tennis, power walking, yoga, weight lifting, etc., at 100% of my previous ability.

What I think as a fitness instructor:

Continuing with or starting an exercise program after breast surgery is crucial to your physical and emotional recovery. Conditioning does not need to be long or intense to benefit you. Taking a brisk thirty-minute walk combined with ten minutes of resistant exercises will increase your energy level and lift your spirits. I have never heard anything to the contrary. So, get up, get out and have some fun!

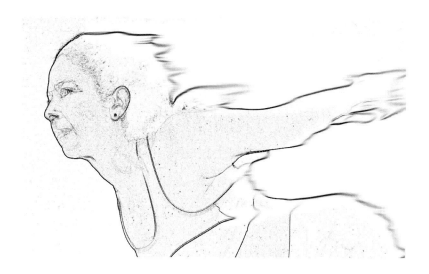

(You never know what will happen when Derek starts getting creative with his own photos...)

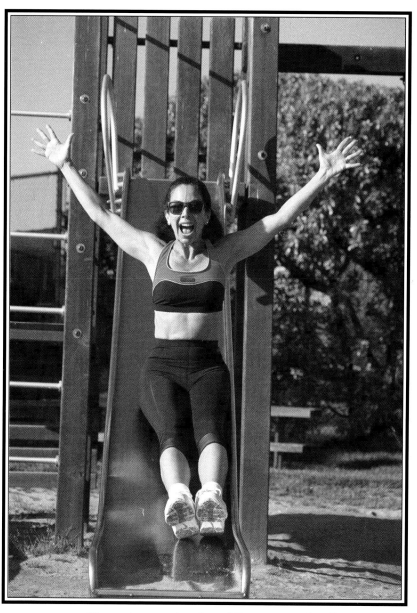

"So, get up, get out and have some fun."

"... I felt then, and I still feel now like I'm supposed to be some kind of messenger, because good breast-cancer-related things keep on coming to me and I'm not seeking them out..."

antoinette galindo

I can STILL have my faith, and I have to remind myself of that all the time.

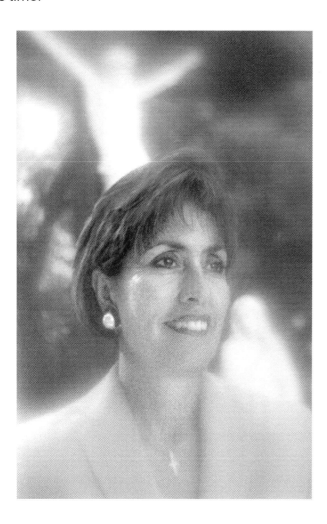

It was just a few days before St. Patrick's Day in 1995 when I went in for a routine check up and a mammogram. My doctor called me the day before I was leaving for New York with eight girl friends and said: "I don't want to alarm you, but we found something on your mammogram that wasn't there before. We should watch it, so in five months we want you to get another mammogram and when you get that done, call me and we'll check it again at that time."

So, I went on to New York, didn't tell any of my girlfriends, didn't think anything more about it. Five months later I went in for another mammogram. My doctor called me right after that and said: "There's still something that I think we should check. We need to do a biopsy." So, without doing any research, I just asked him which surgeon he would recommend, and I went to that surgeon.

I was trying to handle everything on my own, and if I could have gotten away with it, I wouldn't even have told my husband. I just kind of panicked and thought "let's just get this taken care of", really thinking that I wasn't going to have anything, I thought everything was going to be fine, I would have the biopsy, get the results and that would be the end of it. But I had to tell my husband because I needed a ride for the first lumpectomy. I'll never forget how I told him: I was going up the stairs, he was at the bottom of the stairs and I casually mentioned that I just had to quickly go to the hospital in a couple of days… "What are you talking about? What's going on?" he asked. Then he started walking up the stairs, too. I said: "You know, it's no big deal, I need to get a biopsy. 80% of the women that have these biopsies on their breasts get negative reports and I don't think it's going to be anything …

it's no big deal". I was just going on and on… And then he said: "What about the other 20%?" I froze. What threw me was that my husband is a very optimistic person, but when he said that… I didn't want or need to hear that. It was pretty daunting.

I had a biopsy in my left breast in September of 1995. They actually did the biopsy and a lumpectomy at the same time and they found DCIS. After I had the lumpectomy the doctor called and said: "We got it all." I said: "You got what?" " We got all the cancer", he said. All the cancer?… I was in total shock! I had cancer? He said I did, but everything was fine. What would be the next step? He said he'd see me in a year.

So, I had that done and then I went to visit a girlfriend in Aspen and told her what I had just gone through. When I came back from that trip she told me that her roommate in college had died of breast cancer. So, she said: "Antoinette, don't you find that strange? That you had cancer… that you go in for a biopsy, or you think you're going in for a biopsy, and you come out with what looks like a lumpectomy because your breast is smaller. Antoinette, don't you think you should get a second opinion? You have to get a second opinion. What did this doctor tell you?" She thought I should do some research.

I did go get a second opinion. I started researching who the best doctor in our area was and this one name kept on coming up. He worked at a hospital near my home. So I called him and told him what happened and that I wanted to get a second opinion from him. He asked me to send him all my records, but by the end of October 1995 he still hadn't received them. He said they were having a hard time finding my records. He called me in November and said: "They've lost three of the slides to your pathology report, so, we don't know… I can't tell you if all your margins were clear. I want you to come in." It was two days before Thanksgiving, I was having thirty five people coming over for dinner…

My husband and I went in to see the doctor and he said he had good news and bad news. The good news: I was not going to die from this. The kind of breast cancer I had didn't metastasize… the bad news was that, because they lost my slides he couldn't look and didn't know if the margins were clear. He wanted to do another lumpectomy. He said: "I want you to enjoy the holidays, and I want you to come back in January and get this done." And so that was planned and scheduled.

All through this process I really knew I was going to beat breast cancer. I really just had this faith that everything was going to be fine. I did go through some trauma, don't get me wrong. I told my husband and my girlfriend in Aspen, but no one else in my family knew, because my oldest brother had died of cancer at age 44. I was now 44 also, facing cancer, and I didn't want to burden them with my news. But keeping things to myself and internalizing it all wasn't good, either.

So, in January of 1996 I had a second lumpectomy and they found more cancer, but the margins were clear, and after everything was said and done, my doctor didn't think that I needed radiation or chemotherapy, and he didn't put me on tamoxifen, either. I get checked every three months.

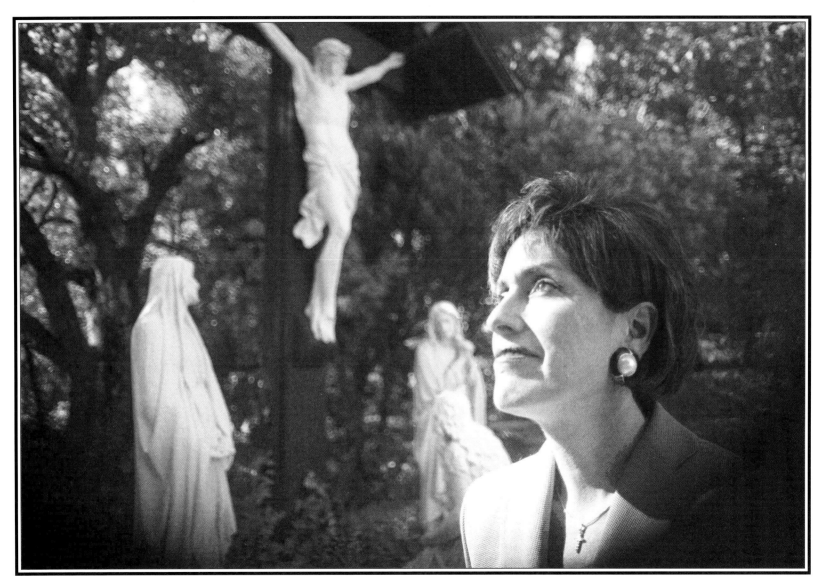

I felt then, and I still feel now, like I'm supposed to be some kind of messenger to other women.

I am now a big advocate of getting a second opinion, because if I hadn't gotten a second opinion, everyone would have just thought that the cancer had recurred, and I wouldn't have known any different. I wouldn't have known that the first hospital had lost some of my pathology slides and I wouldn't have done anything else about it.

I knew God was doing this for a reason. I never questioned why He was doing this or why this was happening to me. I

I knew that someday God was going to give me a reason for all that was happening

just knew that some day He was going to give me a reason for all that was happening. In the mean time I just went about my life. After the lumpectomy I went to work the very next day, I didn't think I needed to give myself time to rest. I noticed that after the surgeries my immune system was out of balance for a while, I caught colds very easily… Today I think it was pretty bizarre how I reacted to all this. And through it all I found that I am a very private person, which I hadn't thought I was before.

In April of 1996 the two hospitals where I had had my two lumpectomies were merging, I filed a formal complaint against the first doctor (the one who did my biopsy and first lumpectomy) because I didn't want something like that happening to another person. I also wrote a letter to the CEO of the second hospital where I had my second lumpectomy commending my new doctor.

Also in April of 1996, my new doctor called me and said to me: "Antoinette, Thursday morning at 11… I have an unusual request." I thought he wanted me to write another letter - he had gotten a copy of the letter I had written and he had thanked me for writing it - he continued: "Would you be willing to go on the Donahue show to tell your story?" I immediately agreed, but soon after that I realized that no one knew about my cancer. I was planning on going on national television to tell my breast cancer story, and no one but my husband and a girlfriend knew about it. Now I was going to have to tell everybody!

While all of this was happening, my face started breaking out and I thought it strange for me to be having acne at that age when I had never had it before. I went to see a dermatologist and after she read my questionnaire she asked what kind of surgery I had had a few months before. She asked how my family felt about my lumpectomies, and when I told her they didn't know, she said: "Antoinette, I don't think you have acne, you're breaking out in hives, you're probably nervous or anxious about your cancer ordeal, you seem to be internalizing it all and that is not healthy. What I prescribe to you is to get into a support group and talk about this, and then tell your family." I thought about my family and my brother again who had died of cancer at age 44, but I followed her advice and went to the support group at the hospital. That's where I met Marianne Riddle and we really bonded immediately. The very first time I was there the floodgate opened, I couldn't stop crying, and everyone at the group was of the opinion that I had to tell my family, even though it was over.

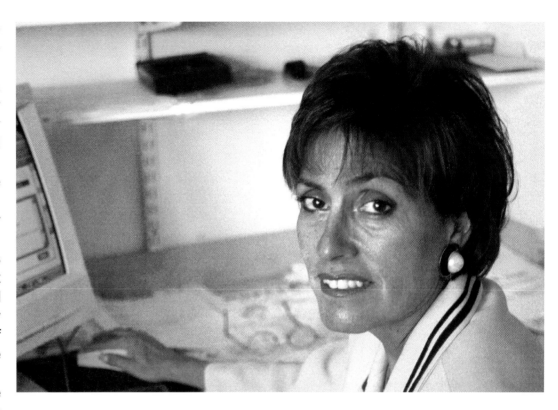

I called my brother and asked him to come to my office. He said: "Come on, Sis, just tell me now." I said: "I had something, but I'm fine now and I don't want you to get all excited... I had breast cancer. I went in... " He interrupted me: "I'm coming over right now." His first question was: "Why didn't you tell us?" I told him I didn't want to worry anyone and that I had thought that had been the best way to handle it.

I hurt a lot of people's feelings by not telling anyone, by not confiding in them, but that's how I usually deal with things.

I asked him to tell Mom - I didn't want to tell her myself - and everyone else in my family, and then I also started telling people. Telling everyone was really something extraordinary because I didn't realize the impact that my-matter-of-fact way of talking about my cancer would have on people... I got notes from my girlfriends saying that I was telling them I had cancer as if I had a cold, as if it was no big deal. But I was confident that I was going to be all right and my faith kept

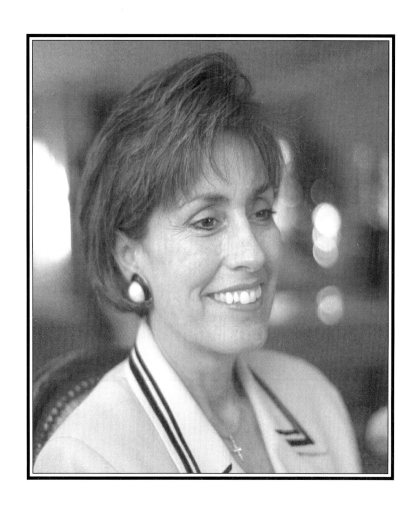

telling me that also. I was going to be all right, and I knew that I was going through this for a reason.

When I was on the Donahue show I told the audience that when you get a cancer diagnosis you have to take matters into your own hands. You have to inform yourself, become knowledgeable about your options and do your own research. You can't be intimidated by doctors, and you should always get a second or even third opinion, if you feel you need it.

After the show, things started snow balling with this breast cancer thing. Someone got my name and through that person I became a mentor at the support group at the hospital where there are so many women who have been diagnosed with my kind of breast cancer. I contact them, talk to them, help them get through their difficult times, and I've talked about my ordeal on the television news as well. I found all of this so amazing and I realized that was my answer: I felt then, and I still feel now like I'm supposed to be some kind of messenger, because good breast-cancer-related things keep on coming to me and I'm not seeking them out. Just like with this book, that I was asked to be part of it, to help others… I've gotten calls from women all over the United States and Canada. People that know about my doctor come out for consultations with him and through the organization, the mentoring program at the hospital they find me, and I help them.

When I was on the television news for breast cancer, a girlfriend of mine, with whom I had lost contact six years before, heard my voice on television as she was washing dishes, so she called me right afterwards. "This is Tina. I just had a lumpectomy, left breast, the same kind of cancer." Here's someone who I hadn't seen for years, with the same kind of cancer. We now talk to each other again regularly. God has answered my question…

I was very lucky, my cancer was caught early, if it hadn't been for the mammography I wouldn't have found out. I realize that I have been fortunate and thank God that I'm fine now. It's a sad reality that we've lost six women from the support group to breast cancer, but it's comforting to know that I have somehow touched their lives. I know I'm one of the lucky ones, but I also feel a sense of helpless, unexplainable guilt because of that sometimes. But, from the very beginning I just knew there was a reason for my having cancer, and I guess God has answered me. For me, in the end He has turned something bad into something good.

Now when I get stressed out I have to put it in perspective because all other little things don't mean anything. I remember my doctor saying to me: "This could totally change your life around." Well, it hasn't turned my life around, but it does make me remind myself of what is really important. It has been an interesting journey.

"... but now I am extremely happy because I am still able to do all the things I love to do."

patricia jednorozec

I can STILL run my life in many different directions by being involved in a lot of things at the same time.

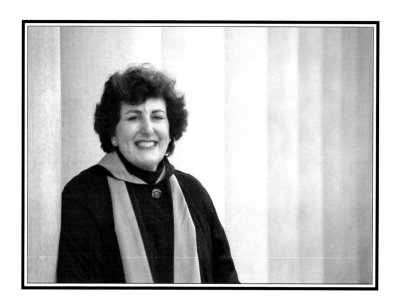

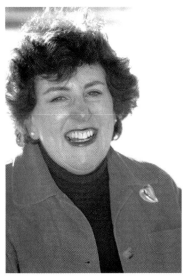

In December of 1991 I was diagnosed with breast cancer. As I was giving my choice of treatment to the doctor, I was very clear that I wanted a modified radical mastectomy. Even though my cancer was very small and had not gone to the lymph nodes, I felt I didn't want to worry about it again. As I spoke to the surgeon, tears were streaming down my face and I tried not to sound as upset as I felt.

On the day of the surgery I said good-bye to my right breast maintaining a sense of humor. As they wheeled me into Operating Room 4, I told the doctor that four was not my lucky number. Needless to say, it made no difference since that was the assigned operating room.

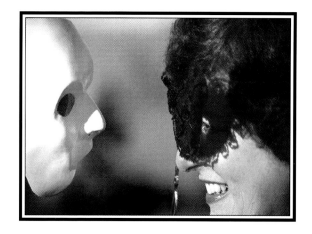

I remember some very lovely people standing there by my bed when I woke up. I remember pressing the button for more morphine to handle the pain.

While I was recovering I read that Erma Bombeck had the same thing. She mentioned that when the lady from "Reach to Recovery" brought her temporary prosthesis, she remarked that it was smaller than the dust balls in her bedroom. That cinched it for me to just be around people that made me laugh. I was in no mood to hear how depressed someone else was about being in this situation. I was feeling that I needed to get my mind off of it, but it seemed that I had to talk about it a lot to get it out of my system.

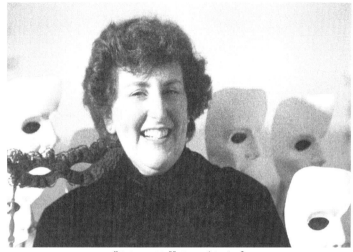

*"I Can Still Run My Life
In Many Different Directions..."*

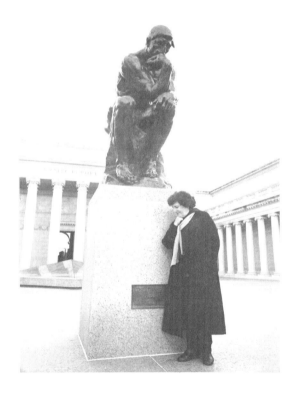

My chemotherapy began on Valentine's Day, 1992, and gave this wonderful day a whole new meaning. The chemo caused me to lose most of my hair, eyebrows and eye lashes, but I handled it with my makeup and filling in the spaces.

My son's Bar Mitzvah was right in the middle of the treatment and that was a good thing because it gave me something else to concentrate on. So there I was, on the day I had been looking forward to, wig and all. I had a great time anyway.

It had been almost nine years and I was faced with another challenge last year. I was diagnosed with Non-Hodgkin's lymphoma. There would fortunately be no surgery, but there would be treatment.

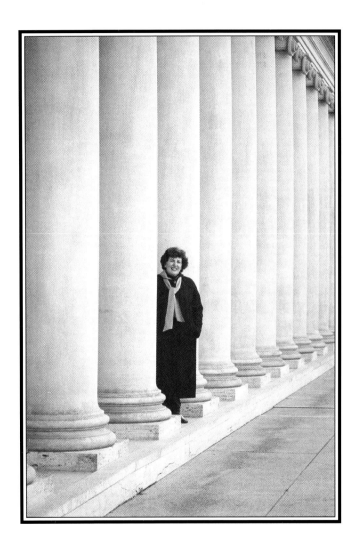

I was given an experimental drug that had been found to cure this disease. After one month after my last treatment - there were only four treatments with Rituxin, one week apart - the doctor said that my CT scan showed a reduction in size of some of the nodules and elimination of others. His plan was to check me every two months to monitor changes.

Today I am extremely happy because I can still do all the things I love to do. I am working as a health education consultant two days a week, as a private practice dental hygienist three days a week, and as a cosmetics company consultant in between. I am able to go back to the gym, and put some effort into cleaning my house. I feel very fulfilled.

It is common for breast cancer to strike families. Very often sisters will be affected, as shown by the inclusion of two sets of sisters among the women in this book.

diana and patricia

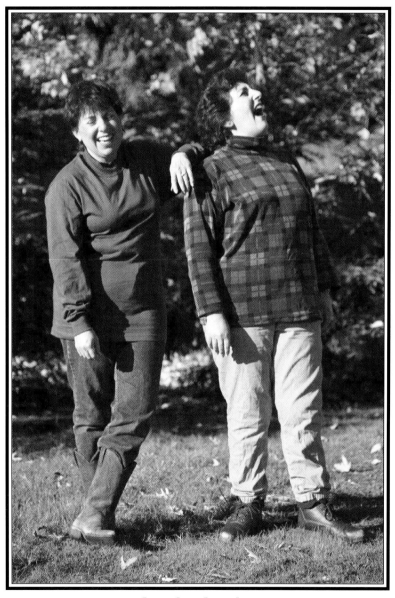

Rebound and Be Alive

"Living each day is so special and making sure you show how much you care for your loved ones is also important."

diana hoffman

I can STILL dance and sing! I can STILL ride my horse...

It was August, 1996 and I was in the process of closing down my law practice that I had successfully had for more than twenty years to start a new venture - one that would make the world healthier, safer and cleaner. I was so revitalized - I would be Chief Executive Officer of a new company called EnviroSystems, Inc. and we would have a new disinfectant that was not only faster in killing bacteria, but also safe for the environment.

I had a mammogram and my doctor called to say that it showed something - I would need a biopsy on my right breast.

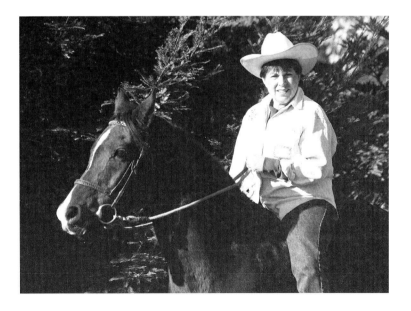

I told my husband and we went to have it done. It was the day before we were moving the furniture from the law office in San Jose to the new company in San Francisco. I decided that the biopsy would not interfere with anything. The next day I was in the office packing, moving things and while not exactly feeling great, kept plugging. My life could be classified as "keep plugging". I enjoy music, horses, and being a part of everything that is happening in the world.

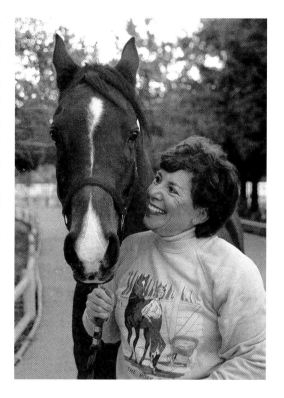

I auditioned for "Camelot" at the Peninsula Center Stage and did not tell them that I would have to have a lumpectomy and radiation. I got in the show that was scheduled to start rehearsals in October. The show was scheduled for 14 performances in December. I would be singing and dancing in the show. A few days before the first rehearsal I had the lumpectomy. Fortunately, a friend of my mother has a house near the theater and I could rest there before the rehearsals.

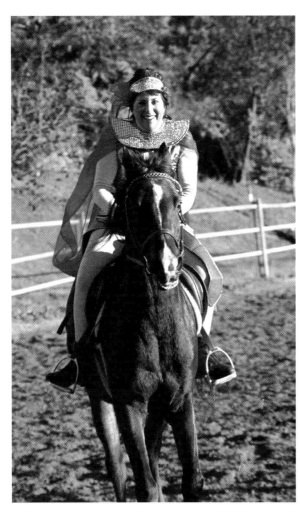

I would go to work in San Francisco, drive to Redwood City to the hospital for my radiation, go to my mother's friend's house and eat and rest for about one and a half hour and then go to the theater to sing and dance until 10 p.m. and then drive twenty miles home. I was able to keep my medical situation a secret from the cast and directors until the third performance when the entire radiation/oncology department of the hospital showed up. The Box Office told the director that about thirty people from the hospital were coming due to my being in the show. The director inquired and I told him. He was shocked. I laughed and said, "I can still dance and sing". Everyone was so supportive and while the production staff was concerned (I think about liability), I dissuaded them by stating that, as "a lawyer", I was assuming my own risk. The show was a big success and it helped me get through a very difficult time, emotionally and physically. It was somewhat like in the "Little Engine That Could" story we read as children. In life if you think you can, you will do whatever you persevere doing.

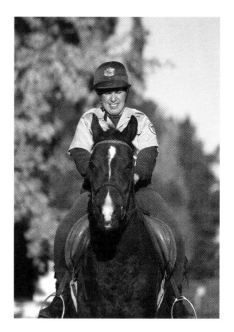

One of the biggest moments during this period was when I finally could get back to riding my horse. I have a wonderful horse I call "Li'l Lucky". He is a registered Egyptian

Rehearsals were every day except Friday nights and Sundays. It was exhausting but it also took my mind off of the discomfort. The radiation oncology department at the hospital where I was having the radiation was amazed that I was doing the show, besides putting in a full day of work from 7 a.m. to 4 p.m. every day.

Arabian that I raised from the age of two (he had been neglected by those who bred him and fortunately, for both of us, I ended up with him). He needed a lot of training and love during the early years and I gave him all that I could, spending the early morning hours with him every day. He is now nineteen years old and we are so bonded.

It was at least three weeks after my lumpectomy when I tried to ride Lucky again. I always mount him from a ledge, since I am only five feet tall, and while he is small himself, it still is easier for me. The first day back I rode him up one of our favorite mountains near Woodside, California. I carry a water container and when we were bounding up a steep incline, it fell out of its holder. I got down to retrieve it and found that there was nothing around for me to climb onto Lucky. I tried to mount him the usual way (foot in stirrup and pulling myself up) but due to weak musculature, I was completely unable to do so. I became very emotional and my sweet horse obviously sensed what the problem was. Without training or coaching on my part, Lucky suddenly put out his right front leg and curled under his left front leg and got down for me so I could mount him. I was so shocked! He had never done that before. I clambered on and wrapped my arms around his neck and just cried for several minutes. He stood quietly (he is usually very spirited and exuberant) and waited for me to sit up. Then he turned and walked slowly down the mountain. When we got back to the stable I told my friends and we all hugged him and cried together. I will never forget this as long as I live. Animals are so loving and understanding - unconditionally.

It has now been five years since the cancer and I am still clear.

I am so grateful to God, my family and friends, and especially to Lucky. Living each day is so special and making sure you show how much you care for your loved ones is also important. I think these are the most important lessons I learned from the experience with breast cancer. Carpe diem is not just a phrase - it is a way of life.

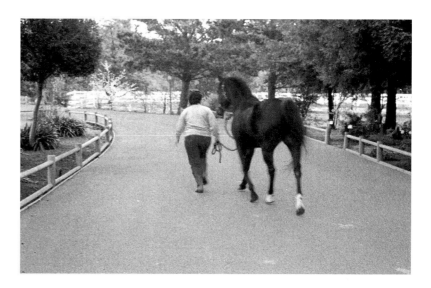

"... I strived to maintain some sense of normalcy within my life despite my illness."

nancy petersen

I Can Still Dream!

On New Year's Day, 1998, I can remember thinking, "This is going to be my year." I was born in '49, I am a San Francisco 49er Fan, and I was going to be 49 years old. But everything changed in April of that year. I was diagnosed with breast cancer. I handled my diagnosis like I did other unfortunate setbacks in my life - I took control of the situation and kept on going. I had surgery, which revealed a medium size breast cancer that had not spread to the lymph glands. Following the lumpectomy, I was treated with radiation therapy and chemotherapy. By October of 1998, I was finished with my treatments. I can still remember dreaming of the day when this would all be behind me so that I could get on with my life.

I did well until June 1999, just around my fiftieth birthday. At that time, I developed diffuse pain in my pelvis. A bone scan showed signs of cancer spreading to numerous bones in my body. The cancer was back, which came as a shock to me as I had negative nodes. The doctors informed me that my cancer was very aggressive, so I once again started on chemotherapy. I went through several types of chemotherapy as well as hormone treatments, searching for one that the cancer would respond to. The various treatments resulted in hair loss, nausea, and fatigue. On that birthday, a friend gave me a card that read, "DREAM - When we take time to dream, we discover the many windows to our soul." Because of the uncertainty of my future, I now had to look at my life,

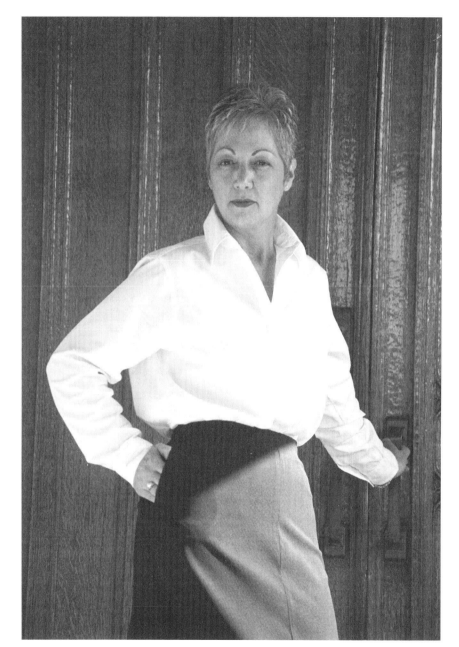

understand what was important to me and choose how to spend each day.

By January of 2000, I was forced to once again undergo radiation therapy to relieve the severe pain I was in. Along with this standard Western Medicine, I used Eastern techniques such as Reiki (an ancient hands-on technique for balancing energy throughout the physical, emotional, mental, and spiritual body) to aid in my healing. After my Reiki treatments, I feel so much better. It takes me to a deeper, peaceful space, beyond the pain. I also use contemplative prayer and meditation to quiet my mind. I rely on prayer for strength and surround myself with peace and enjoy quiet surrender. This helps to bring calmness inside of me and allows me to feel and to just be.

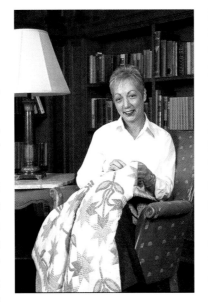

Throughout all this, I still maintained hope, along with courage, strength and spirit. I knew in my heart I was not going to give in to this disease. I managed to keep my upbeat attitude with a generous amount of laughter and my sense of humor. I find keeping a smile on my face, helps to make things a little easier. More than anything, I strived to maintain some sense of normalcy within my life despite

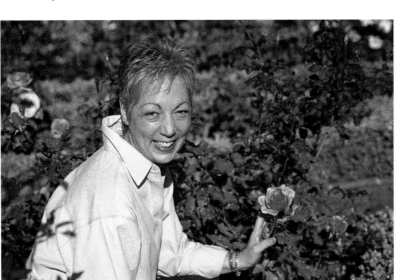

... take time to smell the roses.

my illness. I continued to work full time and remained an active part of my two sons' lives. I was not going to lose this battle. I was not about to give up on my dreams of a normal life.

It was at this time that I began to make some realizations about the way I had been living my life thus far. I realized that I was filling my life by doing for others and not slowing down to appreciate every day. Even though I have an uncontrollable disease, I have been forced to try to control what I can while accepting changes that I cannot. Most of all, I have to take one day at a time, stay positive, and make time to smell the roses.

In May of 2000, I had an opportunity to take a pilgrimage to Lourdes, France. I could have never dreamt that this would become one of the most powerful, the most spiritual experiences of my life. This trip made the events of the past two years fall into place. If you have faith in God you can have hope. My faith has been a source of great comfort and inspiration to me. I know that the possibility of healing goes beyond the

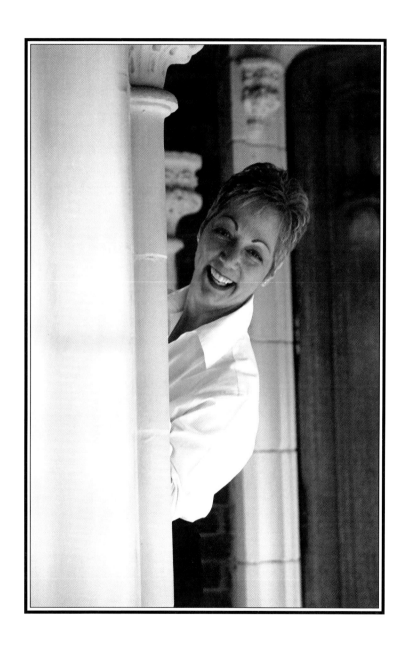

physical and that my future is not in my hands. It taught me to not only accept my disease, but to surrender it to God's will. This ended up truly being a journey of hope and something that I will keep with me forever.

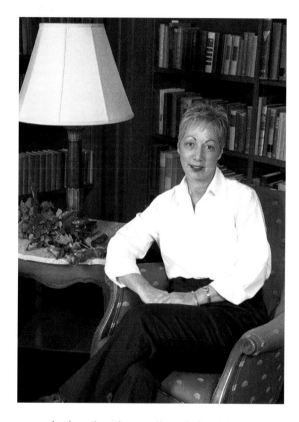

I am happy each day that I am alive. I don't have the energy to waste on worrying about little things. I have realized that life is fleeting and unpredictable and is filled with uncertainty. I have been forced to learn to live in the present and this has been one of the biggest challenges for me. I do have moments of

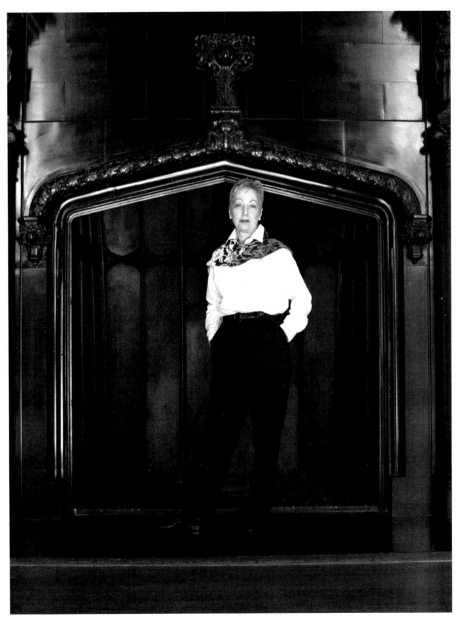

fear, but I have to remind myself to embrace life and live each day to its fullest and to stay open to life's possibilities. I have stopped filling my life by doing for others, and have allowed myself to say NO, which has helped me stay in control of my life.

I have a strong will to live and I will not allow cancer define who I am. I am still a mother, daughter, sister and friend. I still work full time and will continue to do so until I am no longer able. Struggling with cancer has forced me to change my life. It is hard for me to ask for help when I do not have the strength I need to do something, but I now accept willingly. Since my battle with breast cancer, I have learned how to receive love from others and my relationships with family and friends have deepened profoundly. I am so lucky to have these loving people in my life. With the help, love and support of family and friends, I am able to make it through each day.

One thing has remained constant throughout my struggle with cancer. I still dream. I dream of seeing my elder son get married. I dream of hugging my younger son after he receives his high school diploma. I dream of holding my newborn grandchild in my arms. I will not let cancer take away my ability to dream.

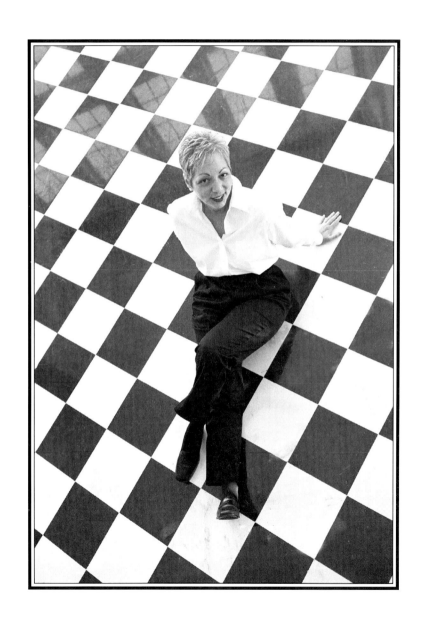

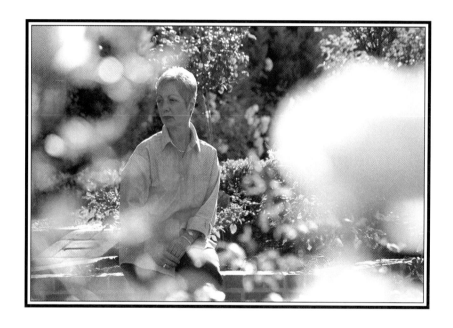

I can still dream

Letter from the photographer

October, 2000

After working on this book for six months I was on a flight to San Francisco to see Aline after she had had a biopsy done on what she had assumed was her "good" breast. It occurred to me then that throughout the book we had been using a term, often also seen in other publications: "touched by cancer". I suddenly realized that cancer doesn't "touch" you, it actually assaults you, it invades you, it disfigures you, it certainly does not touch.

Maybe it is time that we all stop using these "soft" terms to describe something so violent. "Touched by cancer" has now left my phraseology. So, the next time someone you know gets hit by cancer, tell it like it is. It's a long, hard ride to recovery and we have a fight, a battle, indeed a war on our hands. Like any war, to win it takes courage, determination and immense strength. These are the qualities that every one of the ladies featured in this book have displayed. I salute them all.

By the way, dear reader, Aline's biopsy was negative, however the wait for the results was a nightmare for all of us.
Derek

My Mom kept telling me: "We love you no matter what. Not having a breast is not going to change who you are."

maria santiago

I can STILL get up at six and deliver the mail.

I went in for a check up because I could feel a lump in my left breast and it hurt...

"The biopsy report says you have breast cancer and it's aggressive. You have DCIS." Those words scared me, I didn't like hearing them. The days that followed learning about the results of my biopsy were hard to live. I went to the library and read about breast cancer diagnosis and treatment because I wanted to understand what the doctors told me and I needed to be able to know what to talk about with them. My doctor recommended a mastectomy. I didn't really want to lose my breast, so I asked about the possibility of a lumpectomy followed by radiation and/or chemotherapy. He was of the opinion that a lumpectomy wasn't enough because the tumor was at a fairly advanced stage and was of the aggressive type. But it

hadn't spread anywhere and the lymphnodes were all clear and I was thankful for that.

I decided to have a lumpectomy, which was promptly scheduled. I wanted to be awake during the surgery, so I chose to have local anesthesia. I could hear the surgical team talk and discuss what the next step would be, I was able to follow what was happening the entire time. The surgery lasted about one and a half hours, but after about thirty minutes the anesthesia stopped working and I could feel them pulling and tugging. At some point I started to feel the pain as the surgeon worked on my breast, so they gave me more local anesthesia as soon as I told them. The experience wasn't too bad, and I was able to go home soon after the surgery.

Ten days later my doctor called to discuss the results of the biopsy of the lumpectomy and told me that the margins were not clear and that a mastectomy would be my best choice at this point.

I asked the Lord to clear my mind, to help me take good advice from others, to help me think clearly. My Mom was very supportive. She kept telling me: "We love you no matter what. Not having a breast is not going to change who you are, it's only a part of your body. You're married to a wonderful man. Your husband loves you, there is love all around you. We're happy to just have you." But I know it was hard for my mom to find out that I had cancer because she had had colon cancer. She's a very positive and optimistic person, she doesn't sit in a corner feeling sorry for herself or for anyone else, she's a fighter and taught me to be that way also.

I had to make a decision and I didn't want to wait too long. Besides talking to my husband, my Mom and to a few friends, I also contacted a few women at www.breastcancer.com who helped me a lot in clearing things up, answering my questions and giving me support. They talked to me and listened to me and kept telling me not to give up hope. I chose to follow my doctor's recommendation to have a mastectomy.

My doctor talked to me about breast reconstruction a few times and he first suggested a tram flap procedure. I talked to a lot of people who had had it done and they described that it was difficult to make certain movements afterwards. As a mail carrier I thought that type of surgery would make it harder for me to carry the heavy bags. I was almost ready to do it, but then I changed my mind. Then he suggested a saline implant, but I changed my mind about that also at the last minute. I just didn't feel that I needed to have breast reconstruction. I thought that a prosthesis would be just fine and that I could always reconsider the matter at a later time.

I went back to work two months after the surgery. I wanted to give myself plenty of time to recover. Back at work, I started working two hours a day, then slowly increased my hours until I was working full time again.

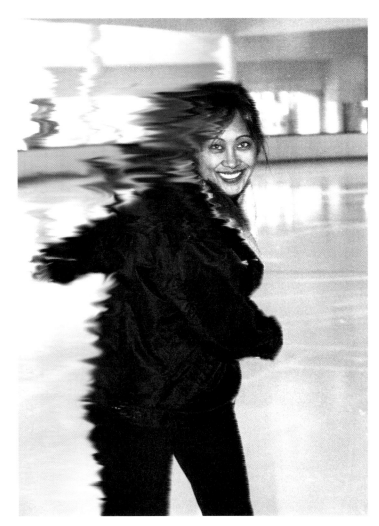

They know me at work as "Sunshine"

I was free of cancer. My doctors didn't think I needed any chemotherapy, radiation or tamoxifen. I had a mammogram on the other breast six months after my mastectomy and it was clean. It seemed that I had a good chance of seeing my daughter grow up.

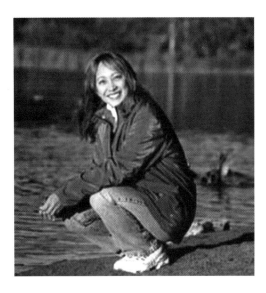

Before the cancer I didn't use to read the bible very often. I was in the darkness, didn't know what to do. Having breast cancer has brought me closer to God and reading the bible gives me a good feeling. My faith is much stronger now. I've learned to enjoy everything, the birds flying, the blue sky and the smell of flowers. Each day is special and life is too short not to be lived to its fullest. They know me at work as "Sunshine".

I can still smile, I can still do everything I did before. I can still get up at six. I am still pumped up about things. I still go out and have fun. Except for my stronger bond to God, I don't know if there is a difference in the way I am. Now, when I think about what happened to me, I realize that I lost only a breast. All in all I'm very happy. My husband still loves me, my mom still loves me, my daughter still loves me. We have no problems with my prosthesis. It's just there, and, as for me, I am just glad and thankful that I am still alive.

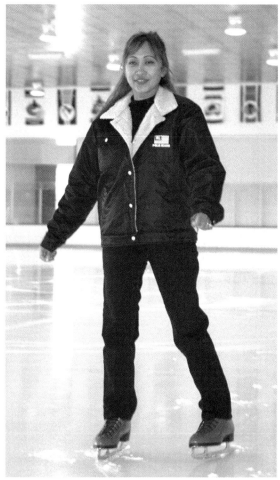

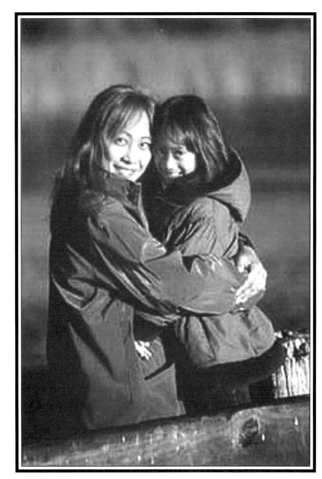

My daughter, my pride and joy.

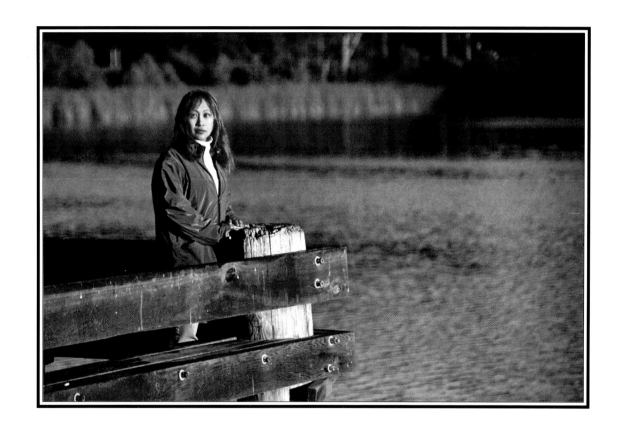

"... My clients and friends would come by the clinic
and would ask to see me: they wanted to see
what look I was wearing."

julieta gonzalez

I can STILL be a vet!

The year was 1996. I was living a very busy life. Running my veterinary practice, and all the hard work that comes with owning a business didn't leave any time to take care of myself. I worked twelve to fourteen hours everyday. At work there were many things that needed my constant attention: clients, patients, surgeries, employees, payroll, taxes, just to mention a few. Outside of work there was my house, my social life and church activities. I had always been thankful and felt blessed for all that I had, but there were certain times when I felt trapped going around and around in a circle.

In September of 1996 I went to my gynecologist for my regular checkup and complained to her of tenderness in my right breast. She said everything was fine, but because I was forty years old she sent me for a standard mammogram that came back normal. In February of 1997, when I returned home to Oklahoma City from a one-month vacation trip - a well-deserved rest - in the Philippines and Japan, I started my activities and hard work again, since my practice was growing very rapidly.

One day in April of the same year I was alone in my clinic after hours, when I accidentally hurt my right breast on a door and I felt an intense pain. When I examined my breast I felt a lump. The very next day I returned to my gynecologist and complained to her about it. She said it was normal and that it

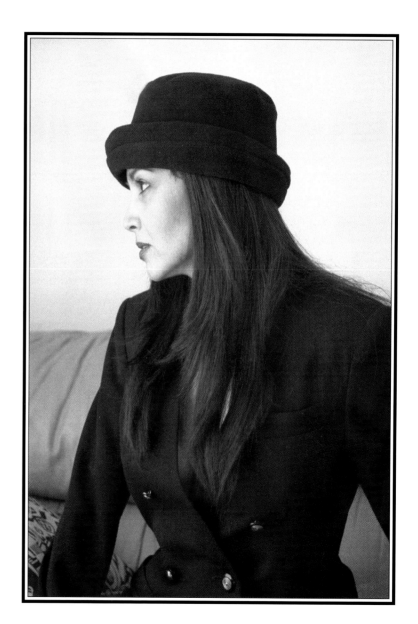

was a cyst. I insisted and told her that it felt abnormal and hard to me, so she sent me for an ultrasound. The radiologist report came back normal and it agreed with my doctor's opinion that it was a cyst. I felt relieved and it also felt as if a weight was lifted from my shoulders because I had kept all this a secret and had not shared any of this with anyone. I did not want to worry my family or anyone else.

In July of 1999 I went to my doctor for a check up and once again complained to her of pain in the right breast in the same place where the ultrasound had showed a cyst two years before. She again reassured me that it was a cyst and told me not to worry, but since it had been a while, referred me for another standard mammogram. By that time I felt something was not right; what I was feeling did not match what the doctor said. Two months before that I had seen a specialist in sleeping disorders because, for the first time in my life, I was experiencing severe insomnia. This doctor, in turn, could not find anything abnormal after a series of tests. I decided to investigate matters on my own and get myself informed about what was wrong with me. I had always been a very healthy person and I was determined to see what the problem was. I knew there was something.

I found out that I was probably experiencing some hormonal changes. I also discovered that there was another type of mammogram called a diagnostic mammogram. I called my gynecologist several times asking her to request a diagnostic mammogram. They did an ultrasound first and this time they did find abnormalities and ran the diagnostic mammogram. I remember it as if it was yesterday: the radiologist showed me the x-rays and told me that my doctor would talk to me

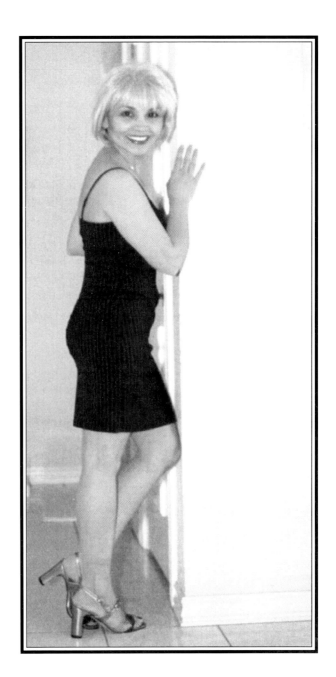

because he was probably not the right person to give me the news, but that the results appeared to be consistent with cancer. I felt a wave of heat rush through my body from my head to my toes and I heard a ring in my ears, but I did not cry or lose my composure. I drove back to work like a robot, not knowing where I was going. I was numb.

After two series of biopsies, one regular and one ultrasound guided biopsy, the definitive diagnosis was made: I had cancer of the mammary gland.

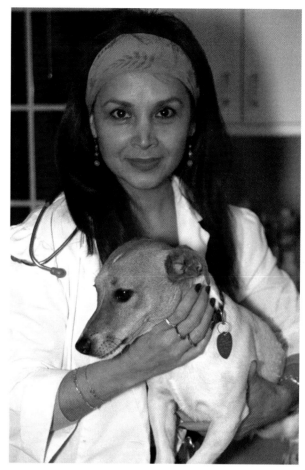

I can still be a vet

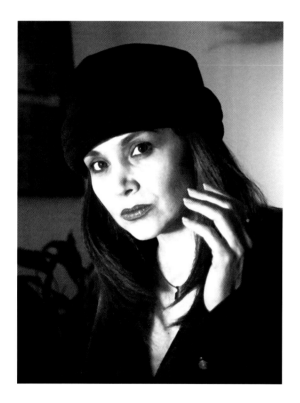

When my family found out, they wanted me to have surgery immediately, but I took thirty days and consulted three different surgeons. I was looking for an experienced surgeon, a breast specialist, one that knew how to use a new technique at the time called sentinel lymph node biopsy to preserve some of my lymph nodes since I wanted to avoid the possibility of

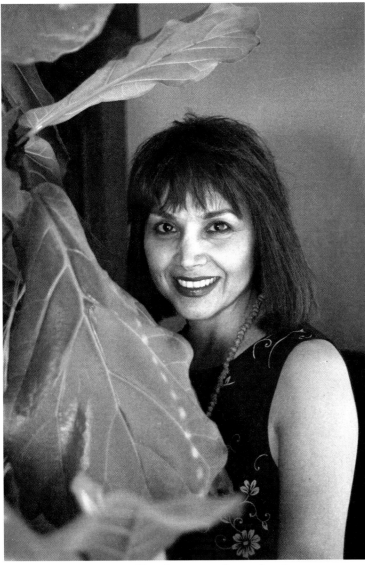
I can still take care of my plants

secondary lymphedema. I also wanted a doctor who was willing to try to preserve my breast. Finally, after some research and with the help of a friend, I found the best surgeon for me. I had surgery on October 11, 1999. I had a quadrectomy and a rotation of my breast to make it look natural.

With the chemotherapy that followed the surgery I lost all the hair on my head and everywhere on my body. First the hair on my head got thinner, then, one morning while I was taking a shower most of it fell off. My sister had to remove it with a pair of scissors since it was all matted and hanging by just a few hairs. I put a hat on and went to work that morning and asked a friend to shave my head to even it out. It was funny because we used the dog's clippers from my veterinary clinic.

The fun part about my cancer came after I lost all my hair. I did not think I was going to wear a hat or a wig, but my friends and family started giving me all kinds of hats, scarves and such things. My sister gave me a brunette wig and then I bought a long brown wig almost identical to my natural hair before I had lost it. Then I got excited and bought a short red hair wig and a platinum blond one. My clients and friends got involved and wanted to see me changing wigs and they gave me five more. Getting ready in the morning became a fun routine: choose a different wig according to my mood and make it match my clothes, make up and accessories, paint my eyebrows and put on fake eyelashes. The platinum wig always looked good with lavender clothes and eye shadow. My clients and friends would come by the clinic and would ask to see me: they wanted to see what look I was wearing.

During that time in my life I felt like I had a license to look any way I wanted. After seven months of chemotherapy I had twenty-eight sessions of radiation to my entire right breast and underarm area and ten more radiation sessions to the affected site. The radiation therapy lasted three months.

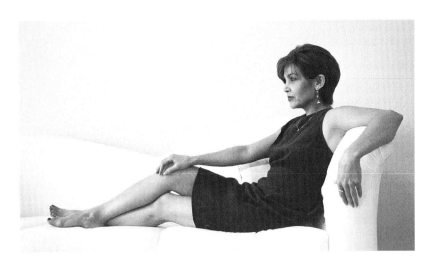

My hair started growing back three months after finishing chemotherapy, but it was different. Before the treatment my hair was straight and now it is a little curly. I still wear wigs once in a while, and I have added a new look with my new curly hair.

I never looked lightly at my illness. It was a long, hard struggle. There were scars and physical pain as well as emotional turmoil and a divorce. But I always kept a smile on my face and no one, not even my family, saw me depressed, sad or bald. I kept those things to myself, in the privacy of my bedroom.

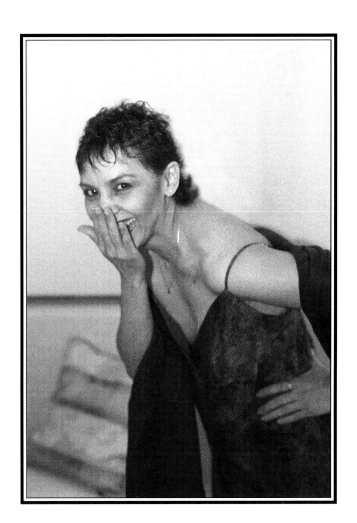

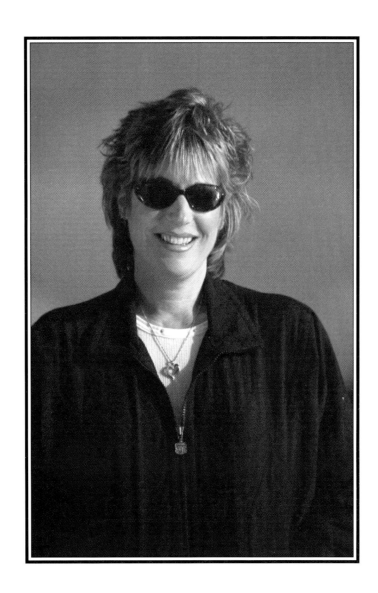

pam thunen

I can STILL laugh! I STILL have a sense of humor!

I am actually a breast cancer survivor twice. I was first diagnosed in 1992 at the age of thirty-seven with a malignant tumor on my right breast, which I found while in the shower. It had gone undetected in my mammogram four months earlier. I tried to pretend it wasn't there, and hoped it would just go away. Obviously, it did not. I had a wonderful surgeon who kept reassuring me that it was probably nothing, since I was only thirty-seven years old, but a biopsy was necessary. Those four days of waiting for the test results were literally hell for me and my family. I could not eat or sleep thinking of the worse. Hearing those words ... "you've got cancer" changed my life forever. I was numb with disbelieve. Why me? I was healthy and young and there was no history of breast cancer in my family. All I could think of was not being alive to watch my two boys grow up, but cancer, as we know now, does not have to be a death sentence.

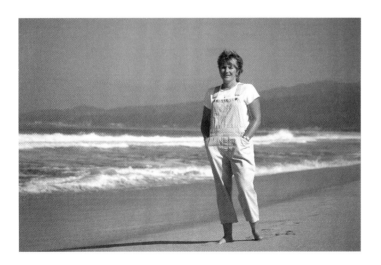

With a lumpectomy and six weeks of radiation I was given an excellent prognosis. I tried to get back to my old life. I went back to work after two weeks and got involved in a support group, which was essential in my healing, both physically and mentally. I developed friendships that I still value. We all have that common bond that no one appreciates, unless you have been there. I began to exercise at the gym, ate healthier meals, took vitamins and began taking time out for me. I was on a mission to get healthy again.

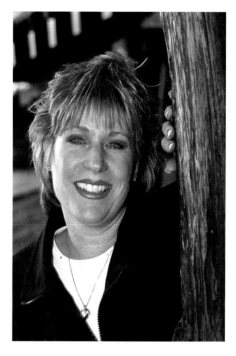

My second bout with cancer came four years later on my other breast, which again was found while in the shower and not in my mammogram. That is how important breast self-examinations can be, they saved my life! I felt this sickness come over me because I knew this time it could be cancer again. What were the chances I could have this awful disease again? This time I wasn't as lucky. The cancer was more aggressive and very invasive. I had one positive node, so the treatment was decided: mastectomy followed by six months of chemotherapy. I have always been a very strong person, but this really took me for a loop.

My sister had been diagnosed six months earlier with the same cancer, same breast, but much more advanced. I was trying to help her cope and be supportive, and then I had to go down the same path again. At least we had each other for support, which helped a great deal. I thought that if my young sister could go through chemotherapy and do all right, then I could, too. As kids growing up, I had always made her go first anyway!

My surgeon sent me to a plastic surgeon for a consultation about reconstruction surgery. He was not only tall, dark and handsome, but also a very nice person. I enjoyed all my visits to his office! Since I was young and very active I decided to have an implant put in immediately after the mastectomy. Everything went fine with the surgery and waking up with some kind of breast was a plus. One step down and one to go. My sister had done much research while going through chemotherapy herself about alternative medicine. She sent me to her acupuncturist who I just loved. I saw him twice a week for almost a year. He had me on all kinds of Chinese herbs along with his treatments. He kept my blood count in balance, so I never needed to skip a chemotherapy treatment. He also helped treat me for my nausea every three weeks. He thought he could help save my hair from falling out, but it did not work. The drugs were much too strong. It seems to me that more and more doctors are accepting the fact that Eastern medicine might be a way to go along with Western medicine of course.

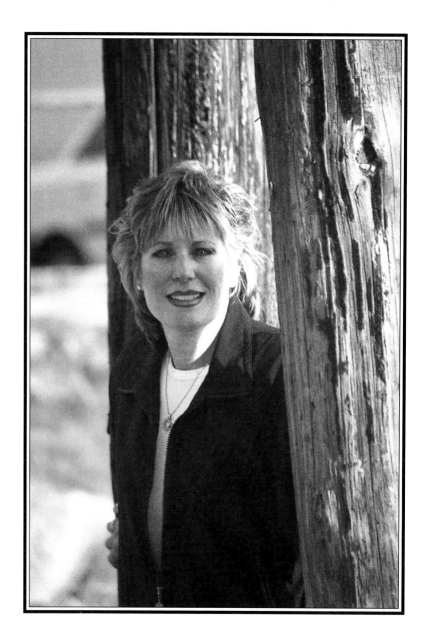

I think losing my hair was just as devastating as losing a breast, although our hair comes back! I found a wonderful wig that looked so similar to my hair no one could tell. I wore fake eyelashes to work and painted my eyebrows. What we do to look good! It was quite a fright looking at myself at night though, but I got over that eventually.

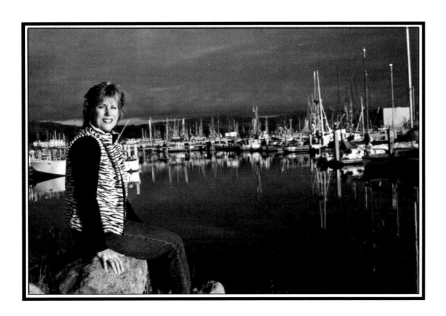

I have a wonderful husband and family that were always there for me. I have two sons that I had to see grow up. They needed their mom as much as I needed them. I am a dental assistant and so I continued to work. I had to keep some normalcy in my life. I have a very understanding boss and very supportive co-workers that helped me get through this rough time. When I felt I needed to go home, I did and went to bed. Being around people that cared about me helped take my mind off this terrible ordeal I was going through.

Six months of chemotherapy done and gone, and I survived it all! It has been five years since my surgery and I have been doing fantastic. My life is as normal as ever, although I look at things a little differently now. I appreciate everything I have in my life. I take time out for me more than I ever did before. My sons are now 24 and 19, and my younger graduated from high school in May of 2001. I really try to put this all behind me now and realize just how lucky I am to have such wonderful and caring family and friends. I could not have gotten through this without them. I kept a very positive attitude during this entire process, which helped to keep my spirit alive. I have been blessed with a second chance at life and I am going to enjoy every moment.

Cancer in northeastern Brazil and the "Espaço Renascer"

The next four women, Maria José, Francicleide, Roberta and Célia are from Recife and Olinda in northeastern Brazil, where I grew up. Medical care and medicine in general are very different in developing countries than in developed ones. In Brazil, cancer is still a disease that is not talked about a great deal, it's a taboo illness, and very often the doctors will not tell the patients that they have cancer, but might, instead, tell one or two family members, usually a spouse or a parent.

Very often when a woman goes in for a biopsy of her breast, she might come out of that surgery without a breast. It is common practice to look at tissue samples while the patient is on the operating table. If the sample is positive, the surgeon goes outside to discuss the issue with the family, makes his recommendation as to what would be best done next (usually a mastectomy). After the family agrees and signs the authorization, the surgeon goes back to the operating room and performs a mastectomy and lymph node dissection. It is quite a shock to most women when they wake up and find out that their breast is gone.

We found these four Brazilian women through the Cancer Hospital in Recife, where my sister, Liliane, also had her breast surgeries. At this hospital they have a place where women can go for support, information, exercise and physical therapy before, during and after their fight with breast cancer. The place is called Espaço Renascer and it means 'a place for rebirth'. As part of the recovery and support program, they have a very artistic, expressive dance, the 'dance of life', that takes you through every step of a breast cancer battle, from diagnosis through the last day of chemotherapy or radiation therapy. It's very dramatic and it has helped many, women cope with this terrible disease. All four of these women have only good things to say about the Espaço and the people that work there. They call themselves "veterans", they have been working there as volunteers helping other women get through their hard times for many years now.

Aline

"... Now, eleven years later,
I am fine, everything is fine...
I feel fantastic!"

maria josé de moura

I can STILL write!

It was April 1990. I was only forty-four. I was having uterine problems and was being treated for that. My gynecologist said I had a myoma, prescribed medication for it and watched me for a while. I didn't see him for a period of time, kept on taking the medication, but the myoma continued growing and I could actually feel it. I was worried and went to see my gynecologist again. He examined me and immediately scheduled the surgery to remove it. It seemed urgent. The day of the surgery they took my medical history, asked about my family and wanted to know if anyone had had cancer. My mother had died of metastatic breast cancer. My lymph nodes had been swollen under my arm for about three years and I was able to feel little lumps in my axilla, but I just ignored them, thought nothing of it. Just before the surgery the nurse asked if I had any skin problems, or if there were any changes in my skin. When I showed her my lumps she went very quiet, told me she would be right back, left the room and came back with a team of doctors. They examined me and wanted to

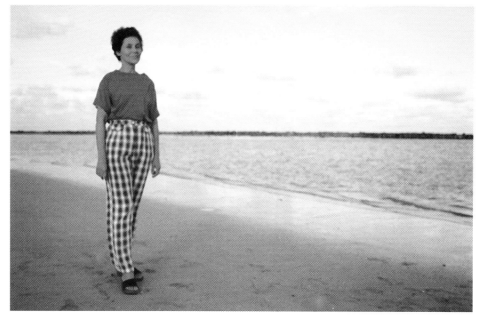

postpone the surgery I was scheduled for, but my doctor didn't think that was necessary. He wanted to go ahead with the scheduled ovary surgery and take the opportunity to biopsy the lymph nodes. I was in the hospital for sixteen days waiting for the results of the biopsy (a long stay like that can be common in parts of Brazil, ed)

On May 7 I had a second surgery to remove the lump under my arm that was already breaking through my skin. It was a large lump, about two inches, but on my skin it looked so small. It was convinced that I, like my mother, had breast cancer, but didn't know about it. The diagnosis: invasive ductal carcinoma. At the end of May the incision was very inflamed and there was only one stitch that looked fine. I went back to the hospital to get the results of the biopsy (it is common practice in some hospital in Brazil to give tests results to the patient who, in turn, takes them to his or her doctor; ed). I took them to my doctor and after he read the report he told me that I needed more surgery. I laughed and asked why. I laughed because I felt so well now. He said: "Maybe I will have to remove your breast, but I will try to just take the tumor out." I think he used the word "maybe" to avoid scaring me, but I think he knew exactly what had to be done.

When he said that I started crying, my life was getting so complicated! Up until now I had taken care of everything related to my disease all by myself, but I felt alone now. I missed my mother and my sisters. The news made me nervous, I didn't want to have another surgery and lose my breast. I wanted to die. I was so scared! My doctor tried to calm me down and talked to me about losing my life versus losing my breast. "What's a breast compared to your life? When you walk on the streets you see so many women without one or even both breasts. There are many of them who have had mastectomies and are now leading normal lives". I cried a lot, but trusted my doctor and resigned to the idea that a mastectomy was the best thing for me, so I signed the authorization for the surgery, which went with no problems. I was told that they had also

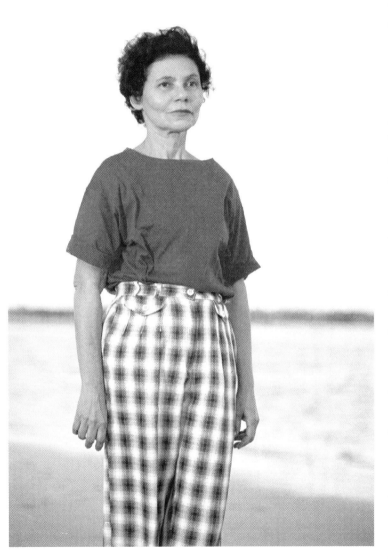

scraped some of the bone off because there was already some metastasis to the bones on my chest. I couldn't believe it. I had never felt any kind of discomfort or pain.

I had more than twenty-five sessions of radiation therapy and five sessions of chemotherapy, one every month, because I felt so sick after each one of them and it took me so long to recover from them. I lost all my hair, was very depressed and upset. At the end of my radiation therapy I broke my arm, it was swollen for two years and I couldn't move it very well. I was told not to use that arm, so, for two years other people cut up my meat for me, peeled vegetables and fruit for me. I couldn't do anything because my arm was so tender and weak, any little thing I tried to do made it hurt. After a while my hands started to become deformed from the lack of use.

Two years after the mastectomy I had twenty-five more sessions of radiation and at some point was told that I needed physical therapy

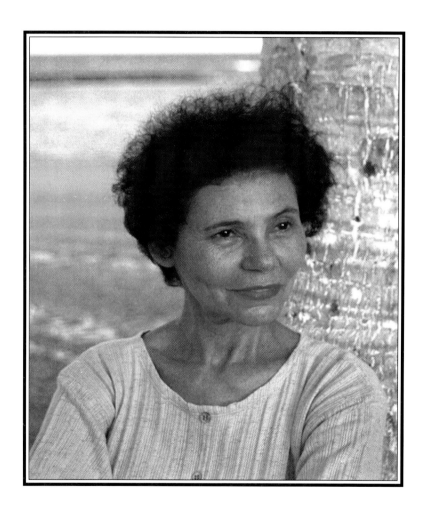

to regain use of my arm, so I was sent to Espaço Renascer at the Cancer Hospital.

The Espaço was a God-sent gift, a light that shined in my dark path. I was so depressed when I went there the first time. I was afraid of doing any exercises, but as soon as I started the physical therapy I started to feel better and get better. After some time at the Espaço the therapist told me that I was a miracle, she had thought that it would be very difficult to help me, but was very impressed with how fast I was getting better. Soon I started taking part in the support group at the Espaço where they work out, dance and talk. One feels so liberated and free at the Espaço. I felt like I had been born again. The Espaço is a place where women who have breast surgery go to give and receive support, exercise and socialize. We have fitness instructors, dance instructors, physical therapists, social workers and psychologists. It is a wonderful place for women at our Cancer Hospital.

We have a dance group at the Espaço. We do a dance called The Dance of Life, and we have performed in several cities in Brazil, both on the coast and inland, and at a few breast cancer congresses throughout the country. There are ten to fifteen volunteer women who take part in the Dance of Life. It is an artistic representation of the steps in dealing with breast cancer, from discovery and diagnosis to the day you're considered "free" of cancer. It talks about self-examination, mammogram, surgeries, recovery, fears and so much more. We all enjoy the part we have in the dance and in the work we do here.

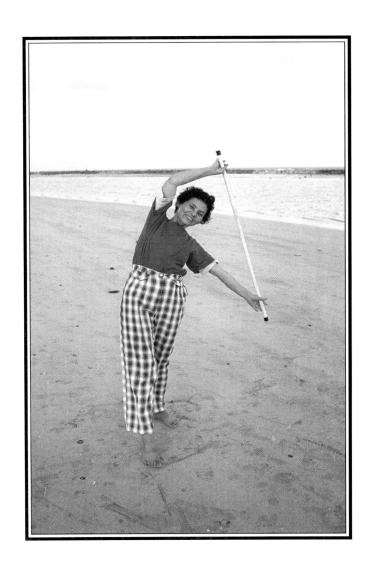

At the Espaço we approach and offer help to newly diagnosed women or to women in treatment who come to us. When they get there they're so down and so afraid. As we support and help them, little by little they start feeling better. Sometimes they comment about their first impressions at the Espaço and how we, the "veterans", laugh and dance. They wonder if they will ever be able to do the same, and some time after they come to us they start joining in and they love it. We are reborn at the Espaço.

I had never danced or done any kind of exercises until I got to the Espaço. There were no physical education programs when I was growing up and I never learned to exercise on my own. Everything changed when I got to the Espaço. As a child, I had wanted to dance ballet, but my family couldn't afford to pay for my lessons, and now, at age forty-six, I started dancing and doing exercises. It was great! My dream of dancing came true after I grew up and because of the cancer. Having breast cancer has changed my life in a good way and in every aspect of it. I used to be sad, pessimistic and depressed. Now I feel young, happy, beautiful, even though I know I'm not beautiful. My recovery has changed my mood and that is wonderful. I am fifty-six now, but my spirit and my mind are only twenty-something. I am open to experiencing anything new and I do so many things now.

I can still do everything I did before. I thought I wouldn't be able to wear my clothes from before the surgery so I gave them away... How silly of me! I thought I was going to die. After the Espaço my attitude towards life changed for the better, I stopped thinking negative thoughts and feeling useless because of my "useless" arm. I do everything myself now. I do laundry, cook, clean my house, just like any other normal person.

My sisters helped me a lot, supported me emotionally through it all. After the surgery I started writing again. I write poems and short inspirational notes. Three days after my surgery I wrote about my doctor, who was an angel in my life. He would come to the hospital where I stayed for two weeks, sit on my bed and read to me. What a wonderful supporting doctor he was! I've written about my stay at the hospital, about going to the surgery, about the surgery, about the Espaço Renascer.

After the surgery I also started singing and I had never sung before. My friend Francicleide took me with her to one of her choir practice sessions and soon after I became a part of that choir, and now I also sing with them. I have a full life: I sing in a choir, I dance the Dance of Life, I volunteer at the Cancer Hospital and now I am thinking about going back to school to take some computer classes. My life has changed and become better.

Now, eleven years later, I am fine, everything is fine. As far as I know and am concerned I am cured. I feel fantastic!

"Cancer has changed my life in a positive way."

francicleide torres cabral

I can STILL sing!

I was only thirty-eight when I was diagnosed with breast cancer. I had just gone back to work at a public hospital after having been at home as a mother and homemaker for ten years. Some people thought I should stop working, but work kept me busy and my mind off of negative thoughts, and I thought that my job would help me recover faster.

I had never felt any pain or tenderness in my breasts, even during my periods. One day I bumped my left breast and felt incredible pain. After that incident my breast became sore and very tender to the touch. But I thought it would eventually stop aching. The second incident happened when I rolled in bed one day and I felt that same sharp pain in my left breast again. I wanted to see my gynecologist, but my husband kept saying it was just my nerves. Nerves or not, I thought I had something and I wanted it checked. I went to see my doctor, but during the examination she said she couldn't find anything, and that I was probably just nervous. I told her I didn't use to feel anything like that before or have any pain, and wanted to know why I felt pain if there was nothing wrong. I asked her to order a mammogram, but she wouldn't, she didn't think it was necessary. I insisted: "Why can't you order one, I'm paying for it, aren't I? I'm thirty-eight, it's time for me to start getting mammograms anyway." I wasn't going to give up until she agreed to send me for a mammogram, which she eventually did, but kept telling me that she didn't think there was anything wrong, that she couldn't feel anything abnormal during the

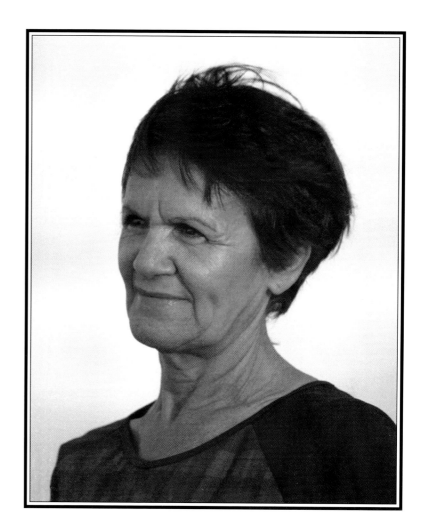

examination. I hoped it was really nothing, but I wanted to know for sure.

So I went and had my mammogram, and, armed with the films and the report, I went to see a doctor friend of my husband's family. After he looked at the films he thought it would be good to have a biopsy done because there was something that probably needed looking at. I had all the required tests done quickly because he wanted to do the surgery that same week. I went back to my gynecologist and asked her to take a look at the mammogram films and the report. She was very apologetic for being wrong.

Going back in time for a moment, when I was single I used to be a professional singer and I also used to work at a radio station reading radio soap operas, which were very popular in Brazil in the past. After I got married I stopped working and became a full time mother and housewife, which was fine for me for a long time.

Someone at the hospital where I worked found out about my job as a single woman and soon after that all my co-workers knew about it also. They were all excited about having an "artist" in the staff and were all of the opinion that I should go back to singing again. But I didn't really think I could, I hadn't sung in over ten years. That was when the directors of the hospital told me about the hospital choir. I had never sung in a choir, but singing again would be so nice. They encouraged me to go for an audition; it wouldn't hurt to try. I would be able to practice two days a week during work hours. So I went to see if I could get an audition, which went very well and got me an invitation to join the choir and start practicing as soon as

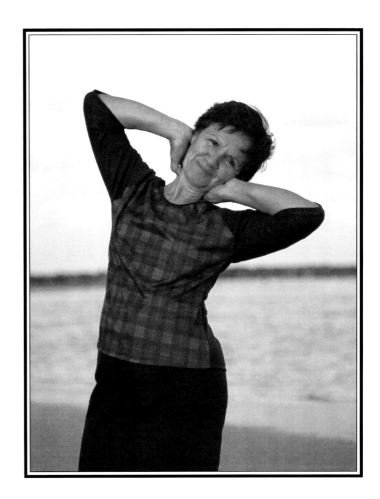

possible. My life changed. Things snowballed from there and I started singing again at weddings, wedding anniversaries, birthday parties… I got quite a few gigs!

The amazing thing was that my joining the hospital choir and discovering I had breast cancer happened in parallel. I was very excited about singing again; my husband and everyone in my family were giving me a lot of support both in my battle with cancer and in being part of the choir. I think the combination of my family support and singing again really helped speed my recovery and keep my spirits up.

My surgery was scheduled for what I thought was going to be the removal of a lump, but I was told they had removed my left breast the day I was released from the hospital. I was in complete shock when I heard they had taken my breast. Why? It was just a lump! No one had discussed the possibility of losing my breast with me. I was told that they had removed the breast because they wanted to prevent the same thing from happening to the right breast. They specifically told me that I did not have cancer, that there was a lump that could have become cancer and they wanted to protect the other breast. They also didn't tell me about the lymph node dissection… I found it so strange that my left armpit looked so sunken.

Things happened that way because I didn't know anything about breast cancer diagnosis or treatment. I was completely ignorant about all of it. I just blindly trusted the doctors.

I learned about the Espaço Renascer when I was going through radiation therapy. The doctors at the Cancer Hospital often send women who have breast surgery there to start exercise programs to help with recovery and to educate them about lymphedema and other things related to breast cancer. I retired in 1995 and started going to the Espaço Renascer. My left arm swelled a little, but with time, exercise and the help of the fitness and health experts at the Espaço, it went back to normal and I also lost twenty-five pounds in the process. I am a very active participant in the Dance of Life. I've been doing it for many years now. I love it.

I didn't have breast reconstruction. I wear prosthesis and I feel good about that. When I started going to the Espaço Renascer, I heard from several doctors who go there to educate women, that breast reconstruction was always an alternative for anyone who wanted it. But, not having a breast didn't bother me then and doesn't bother me now; my husband still loves me and is still attracted to me. I could have done it, the insurance would have paid, but I didn't really want to have any more surgeries, and my life was full of good things: I was singing again, I had a nice job, a wonderful husband and kids. I was happy just like that.

As the first few years passed after my surgery, every so often my husband would ask me: "France, how long has it been since your surgery?" I didn't understand why he asked that sometimes. Then one time when the question came up in conversation again I wanted to know why he kept on asking me that. All he said was that, "as each year passes, we know that you're getting better." At around the sixth anniversary of my surgery he asked me one more time: "It's been five years since your surgery, right?" When I told it was actually almost six years he said: "Thank you, God!" Why? I didn't understand.

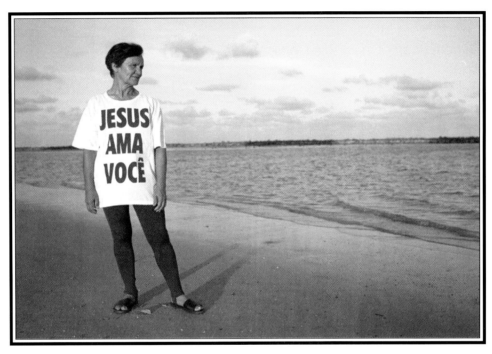

Jesus loves you!

That was when he explained to me that, six years before, the doctor had told him and his mother that I had indeed had cancer in my breast. They were told that it sometimes reccurs within five years. As the years passed and I didn't have cancer again, my chances of having survived it were very good. I can only imagine what it must have been like for my husband and mother-in-law to keep that information from me for almost six years. I understood my husband's question then.

Now, what neither of them knew was that I had known it had been breast cancer all along. As an employee of a hospital, you learn to understand the words the doctors and nurses use. I got very curious when they gave me the paper work to start my radiation therapy. I managed to get my hands on the code book and simply checked what that number on the therapy order meant: 174, breast cancer.

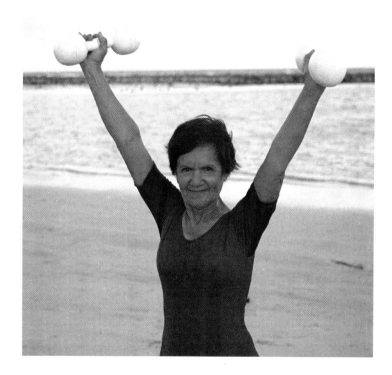

All that happened a long time ago. I am thankful to God that I have been cured from cancer. It hasn't come back yet and I've had no other problems. I am fine now and I can still sing to this day. Cancer has changed my life in a positive way.

"I have stopped worrying so much about material things and learned to value and be thankful for what I have..."

aldira roberta de oliveira

I can STILL enjoy the beach, my favorite place on Earth!

I am originally from Garanhuns, a small town in northeastern Brazil where there are no universities, so I moved to Recife because I wanted to go to school and become a pharmacist. I had worked at several pharmacies for many years and wanted to have one of my own some day. After a lot of hard work I finally achieved my goal and for ten years was very busy . Although my husband and one of his nieces helped me, I opened and closed the business, worked very long hours every day and, therefore, didn't have much time for too many things besides work.

One day in the shower, I felt a lump in my breast. It didn't hurt, so I didn't think anything more of it. A little while after that I was in casual conversation with one of my clients when I told her about the lump I had felt. She immediately became worried and advised me to go see a doctor as soon as possible. She kept saying that this might be something serious and that I probably

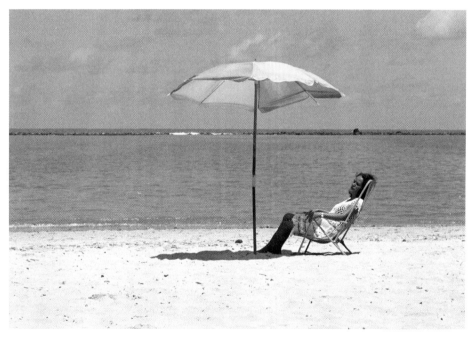

should have it checked out. She mentioned that there had been someone in her family that had found a lump in her breast, just like I did, ignored it for a long time and when it was finally checked out, it was too late.

At this point in time, business at the pharmacy was slowing down, I had a lot of late bills, and I worried constantly about everything, including the lump in my breast. I thought it was a good idea to follow the client's advice, made an appointment to see a doctor, and a surgery date was scheduled. I don't know if a biopsy of the tissue taken was done or not. When it was time to remove the stitches I went to the Military Hospital near a pharmacy where I had worked once because I didn't want to go back to the hospital where I had had the surgery done. The doctor at the Military Hospital told me to go back and see my doctor because, in his opinion, the area where I had the lump still felt hard and lumpy.

When I went back to my doctor he said: "Yes, it does look like you still have a lump in your breast. We need to operate on you again." I was in total shock! I explained to him that I had no time for this, that

I worked very long hours, that I had my own business and it demanded my attention from morning until night. I asked him: "How can this happen? I didn't even know I had two lumps." I took a cab home; I was devastated. I didn't want to go back to see him, so I went to the Cancer Hospital. The doctor who saw me there told me I needed surgery as soon as possible. He said that I had a very large tumor, called three other doctors to examine me and soon after I was scheduled for a biopsy.

I became very nervous and depressed. I was crying as I waited for my turn to go to the operating room. I remember my doctor trying to cheer me up by saying that he would not operate on me if I continued crying like that. So they took me to the surgery room, took some tissue out for a biopsy while I was under anesthesia. The result: positive for breast cancer, DCIS. The doctor went outside to talk to my family and my sister who were in the waiting room, explained to them what they had found and told them that he wanted to perform a mastectomy. He needed the authorization from my family to do that, since I was under anesthesia, they agreed to the mastectomy and when

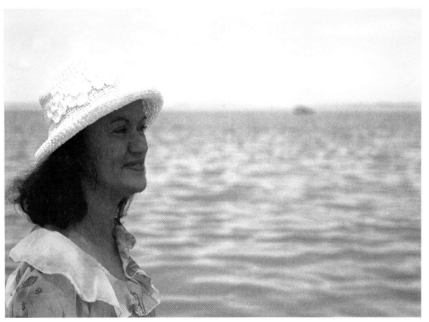

I love the sea, the beach...

I woke up from the surgery my left breast was gone. I remember that day so well: March 7, 1995. After the surgery I had radiation therapy for a while and took tamoxifen for four years.

I went back to work at the pharmacy as soon as I could, but later decided it was time to sell the business, pay my debts and live a more relaxed life - the doctors had told me that stress and emotional turmoil might be contributing to my cancer. I got a job as an employee at a pharmacy near my house where I have been for four years now.

In April 2000 I started feeling pain throughout my left leg and in my bones. I was, of course, very worried, so I went to see my doctor and asked her to please check. I wanted the best test available because it was very painful and I was afraid it could be metastasis. The bone scan confirmed my suspicions: metastasis in the spine. I had radiation for a while.

In September 2000, because my ovaries had been affected by the tamoxifen, my doctor recommended doing a hysterectomy, which was done and from which I recovered without major problems.

In January of 2001 I was checked for metastasis again

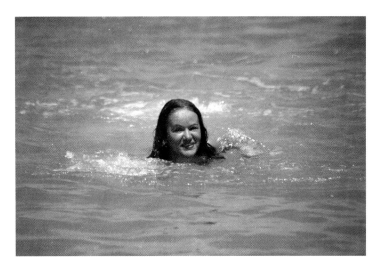

and all tests came back negative. I was told that everything seemed to be fine and was congratulated on my recovery. I was prescribed a calcium supplement that I still take regularly. I like to think I am cured. I thank God and my friends who prayed for me. I think it was their prayers that saved and cured me. I am a more relaxed person now.

Today, I've gone back to work, but I don't work as much anymore. I have sold the pharmacy because I was the only one truly taking care of the business. My husband was also my business partner, but he wasn't involved in helping run the pharmacy very much. I used to work too much because of being responsible for everything, which I still do today at home, but there's no business related stress anymore since I sold it.

I have my God, my sister and my friends to thank for helping me get through my cancer battle. I am generally a happy person, and after the surgeries, I started appreciating myself

more, I stopped worrying so much about material things and learned to value and be thankful for what I have. I have plans to travel and visit places I've always wanted to visit, I have plans to enjoy life, live a more relaxed, fulfilling life, after all I am only forty-three and I have the rest of my life ahead of me.

I have recently visited Aldeia, a beautiful, rural area near Recife. It was a wonderful trip and I truly enjoyed the beauty of Aldeia: the luscious green trees, the walks in the woods, the silence, the peace of watching the animals. I was pleased to check that off my list.

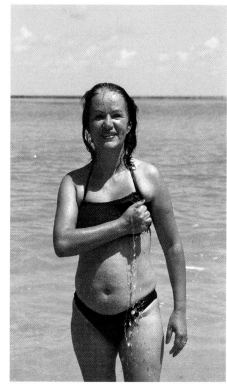

Today I can still do all the things I used to do before the cancer. I love the sea, the beach and nature in general. My passion is going to the beach and now I go to the beach twice as often as I used to. Sometimes, when I'm not too busy, I go every day and immerse myself in the peace and quiet that the ocean gives me.

Yes, I wear my prosthesis even when I go to the beach, and it does get soaked.

"... Life goes on;
you can't let bad things get to you..."

célia muniz de lyra

I can STILL go crazy during carnaval!

I'm seventy now. I was born in Olinda, grew up in Olinda and I adore Olinda. I do, and have done for many years, volunteer work at different hospitals in Recife and Olinda. I work with the poor, the elderly, the leprous and the mentally disabled at these hospitals. I love my volunteer work, I love being able to help care for others and that, in turn, helps me get through my own crisis in a positive way.

I had my mastectomy in 1988. I was in Paraguay when I felt something might be wrong with my right breast. My sister-in-law, who's a doctor, checked me and said that it would be a good idea to go see my doctor back home in Brazil. After returning home I saw my doctor who, after examining me, said she could find nothing wrong, that it was probably my nerves. I went to get other opinions and they all said the same: "there's nothing wrong with you". But I was worried, and finally one of the doctors I saw ordered a mammogram so I would stop worrying and relax. When he saw the mammogram film he said it was just some common calcification, which was common in women who never had children. He was of the opinion that it was nothing to worry about.

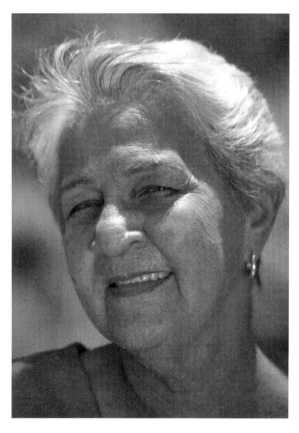

On Monday I went back to the hospital where I worked as a volunteer and started talking to one of the doctors about my mammogram. I had my films with me and he asked to see them. He looked at them and then examined my breasts. It was painful when he touched this one area in my right breast. He wanted to do a biopsy immediately, so I was told to start the process of checking into the hospital so they could start running some tests before the surgery that he wanted to do that week. Well, the surgery posed a few problems because I had and still have a few other health problems: diabetes, heart problems and high blood pressure.

So the necessary tests were done and on Thursday I had my surgery. My husband and my family were there, but no one really worried because we all thought it would be nothing. My cardiologist was also present during the surgery, in case they needed him. Of the five sample tissues they took and looked at as I was still on the operating table, four were highly aggressive breast cancer. The surgeon wondered what they should do next considering my age and my other health problems. My cardiologist told the surgeon that I was a strong person and gave the go ahead to perform a mastectomy after consulting with my husband and my family waiting outside.

So they did the lymph node dissection and a radical mastectomy of my right breast. When I woke up from the surgery, I wondered where I was, where my husband and family were and what had happened. I was under the impression that they hadn't even started operating on me yet. So the surgeon told me what had occurred in the operating room. I remember being upset, but not really shocked. I'm a very positive person, and I remember saying to myself that it was only a breast they had taken, not my arm or anything else. I also told them to take whatever else they had to as long as they took all the cancer. I had a lot of support from my husband, my doctors, my co-workers, my family, and from all the women at the Espaço Renascer.

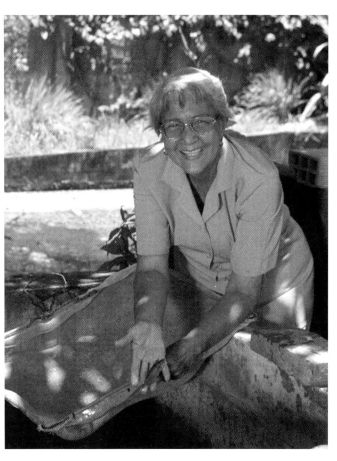

After the surgery things were fine, although I was uncomfortable because of the diabetes and high blood pressure. The doctors were watching me closely. Shortly after my surgery, my sister, the only sister I had, had a fatal heart attack and that, as you can imagine, was devastating.

I chose not to have reconstruction and wear a prosthesis. As I recovered from the surgery I was very worried that my husband wouldn't like me anymore. On a conversation we had and that I will never forget I told him that my breast was gone. His words to me were: "Célia, I married you not because of your body, but because of your internal beauty, because of the feeling of security you gave me, because of the love that existed and still exists between us, because of your wonderfully upbeat personality, because of your honesty and love you have towards other people... Your not having a breast doesn't come into the equation." The subject was never brought up again. We understand each other and we have never had big problems. I love him.

Life goes on, you can't let bad things get to you. I truly believe that when one door closes on you another one opens somewhere else. At the hospital where I volunteer the most, sometimes I'm called to see someone at the breast surgery wing where there are women of all ages who need someone to talk to. They cry, don't know what to do next, are so upset! They tell me that I can't understand what it's like to lose your breast... that's when I just pull up my blouse and show them my scar from my mastectomy. They see how upbeat I am about life and other things, and slowly feel better. I love that part of the job!

Dancing is my passion, I love to dance, especially during carnaval. I love working as a volunteer at hospitals, I have done that since I was a girl scout, and now volunteering at hospitals has become even more meaningful for me.

At the Espaço Renascer I took part in the Dance of Life for a while, but it got me depressed every time I did it because I relived the same excruciatingly detailed diagnosis through recovery steps constantly, and that kept me from moving on, so I quit doing that.

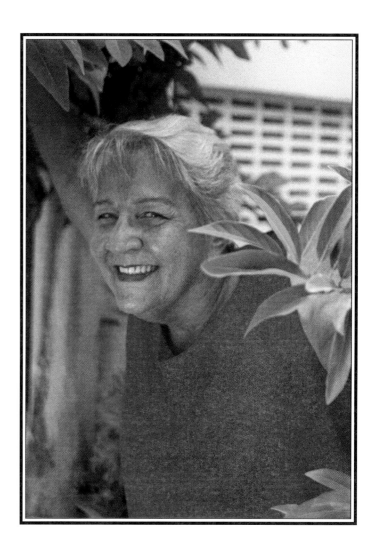

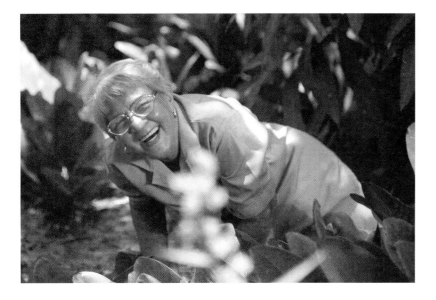

I am a happy person. I am happy now and I thank God that I didn't lose a leg and so, and that means I can still dance. I could have lost an arm or my vision. It could have been worse.

"... My bonus miracle came a little more than two years after my breast cancer diagnosis... the birth of my son..."

bonnie foster

I can STILL enjoy the miracle of Christmas!

Christmas holds an extra special meaning for me. As I celebrate the miracle of God's gift of his son to the world I also celebrate the miracle God has granted me. I was diagnosed with breast cancer less than one week before Christmas in 1993. I was thirty-three years old. My cancer was diagnosed at a very early stage. Despite my physician informing me that breast cancer detected in women under the age of thirty-five tends to be quite aggressive, mine was not.

"For God has not given us the spirit of fear; but of power, and of love, and of a sound mind" (Timothy 1:7). This

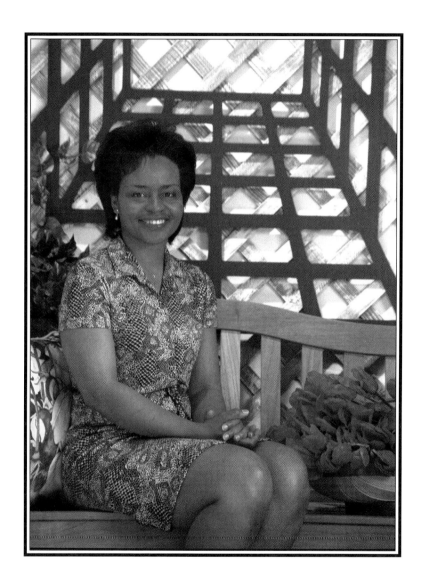

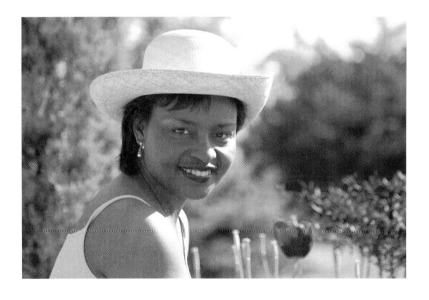

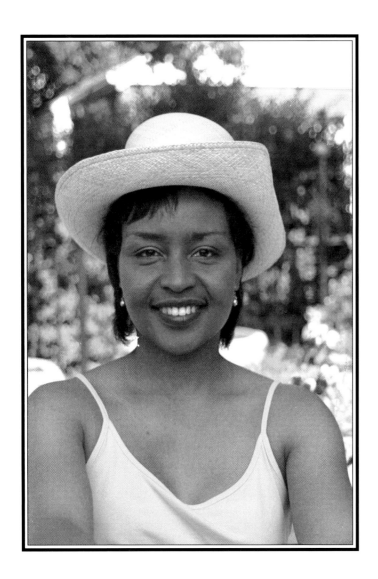

scripture sustained me through the numbness and shock of my diagnosis, the tedious process of making decisions about my medical treatment, as well as my recovery from breast cancer surgery. The scripture also expresses my hope that all women would use a sound mind and not be victims of fear concerning breast cancer. I would hope that all women be aware of risk factors for breast cancer and be even more aware that over 60% of women with breast cancer fall in no high risk categories. I would hope that all women would use a sound mind and perform monthly breast exams, as well as have annual mammograms as directed by their physicians.

After undergoing breast cancer surgery I have been cancer free. My bonus miracle came a little more than two years after my breast cancer diagnosis. That miracle was the birth of my son, which came exactly two years to the day of my being released from the hospital after surgery. God has blessed me beyond measure and I am eternally grateful.

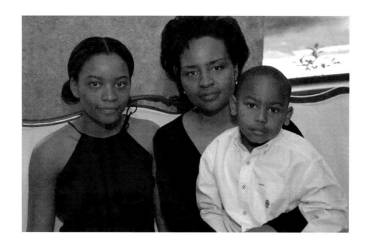

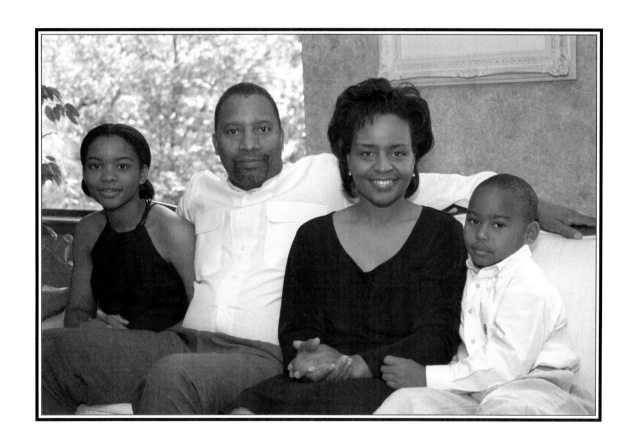

"I thank God everyday for my second chance in life"

brenda c. paxton

I can STILL be a teacher!

I am a thirty-four year old wife and mother of three children. I was diagnosed with breast cancer in the spring of 2000 when I was thirty-three years old. I had a mastectomy in March and chemotherapy for six months. It has been five months since my last chemotherapy treatment. I still think about cancer everyday, but I will not allow those thoughts to control my world. I am doing well and I thank God everyday for my second chance at life. I live my days with a positive outlook on the future. It is a joy to watch the sunrise in the morning and the sunset at night. I have a whole new outlook on life and I don't worry about the little things anymore. I just want to enjoy every minute with my family and friends.

I would like to speak to those who perhaps have just found out that they have cancer, or they may be going through cancer treatments. I want to tell you to keep your spirits up, and keep the faith. It is so important to let your family and friends help you through this difficult time. I know that can be so hard at times, but you need their help, love and support. I would like to say: Don't give up on your dreams. They can still come true.

I have not given up on my dream. I attend college at University of Central Oklahoma, in Edmond, Oklahoma. I am majoring in Early Childhood Education. It is a great privilege for me to walk across the college campus, or sit in a classroom. I look forward to being responsible for my own

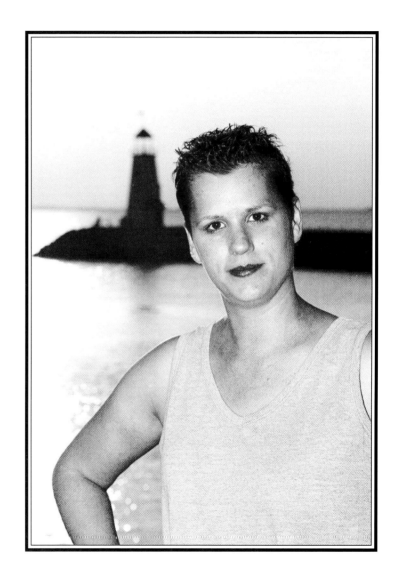

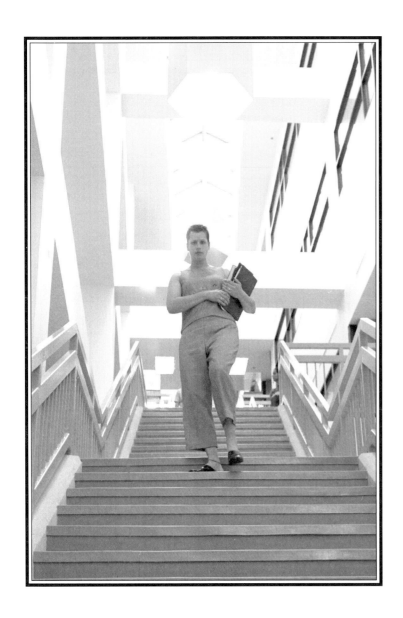

Kindergarten class. I know my year-long experience fighting cancer has made me an even stronger person. I have become more compassionate about life. I have learned a tremendous amount of patience. I believe all of these qualities will help mold me into a great teacher.

I would like to talk about my husband, the person who has been by my side through this whole ordeal. I cannot imagine having shared this experience with anyone else. Scott has showed me more love and support in the last year than some people will ever experience in a lifetime. We have cried together, yelled together and laughed together. I know he will always take great care of me and of our children. He is my heart and soul, and my best friend. My husband and my children bring great joy to my life. I cannot image life without them.

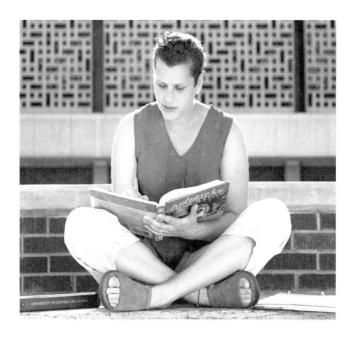

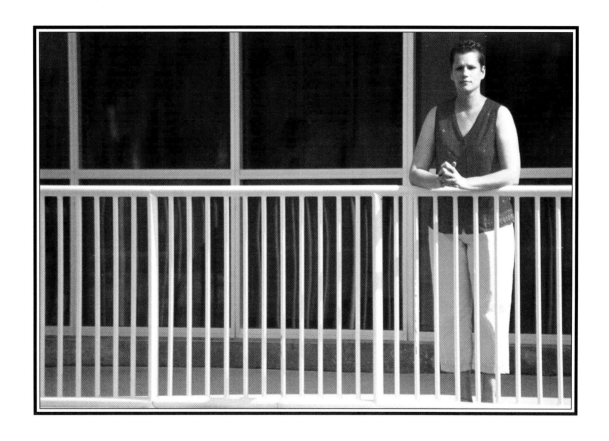

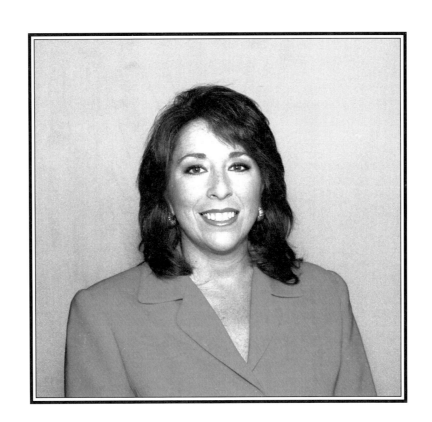

cherokee ballard

I can STILL deliver the news!

In the fall of 1998 my young thirty-five year old body started experiencing extreme pain and fatigue. I thought it was my diet ... and my rough work schedule. I am a news anchor and reporter for a very competitive station in Oklahoma City. We work ten hours a day on average, traveling the state, sometimes staying overnight in places no one should go, all in search of that next story.

I was healthy, I thought, and physically in good shape, but the pain would not go away, pain in my chest like I had never felt before. I thought I had pulled a muscle in my right arm and chest. My doctor didn't believe me, so he pumped me full of pain pills and muscle relaxants and at one point suggested anti-depressants. This went on for about ten months, to the point one day I could not walk up the stairs at my condo. I knew something was wrong one night lying in bed when I felt something move in my chest. I knew something abnormal was in there, something that should not be moving around and growing with each passing day. I had seen the doctor a number of times and he never took a blood sample, never took an x-ray, he did nothing. So, I called for an appointment. This time I got mad. I cried and he told me I was being "fatalistic".

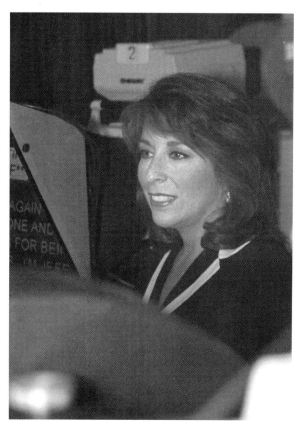

No kidding! He had no idea how close he was to being correct on that diagnosis. I could have died. Once he finally took me seriously, he sent me for a simple x-ray. There it was, a tumor as big as a grapefruit in my chest. That was in the summer of 1999. Next step, a biopsy and it turned out to be cancer: aggressive Non-Hodgkins Lymphoma. I know that, unlike the other women in this book, mine wasn't breast cancer. But because it was in my chest, many people thought I had breast cancer. I didn't. But cancer of any kind is scary as hell. You automatically think: Death Sentence.

So, the diagnosis made, I met my oncologist who said quite honestly I had an 80% chance of survival. I liked the odds, but didn't like what was to come. I had six rounds of chemotherapy called CHOP and total of twenty radiation treatments.

Those were daily and I managed to get through all of the treatment with very little discomfort. I, of course, lost my hair, which was devastating. I bought wigs, which was fun, and lived my life like other cancer patients. The worst

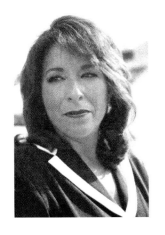

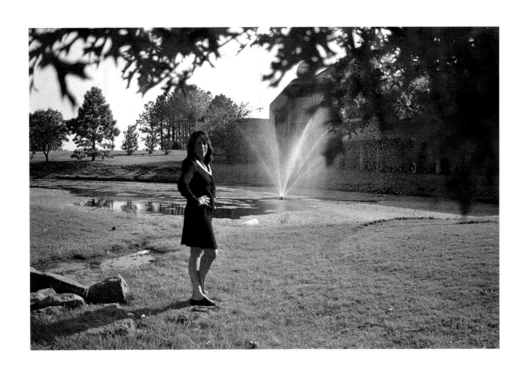

"... I have
a lot of life
left to live."

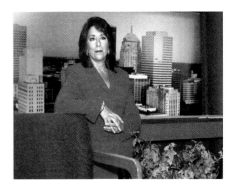

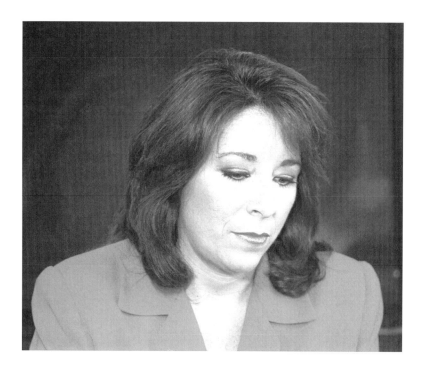

I live each day differently than before. Some relationships changed, some improved. I am much more thankful to God for helping me survive and I love my family more than before. Most of all I thank everyone who prayed for my successful trip through this awful disease. It's horrible and it attacks every part of your body and soul, but I'm a better person for it. I believe I got cancer to change my life and it has. For that I'm thankful, and continue to live (fingers crossed) cancer free. My doctor tells me that, at this point, I'm cured. I still pray daily that the cancer never comes back. I have a lot of life left to live. I'm too young to let this disease kill me. One thing that will always haunt me is not knowing where it came from, how I got it. It's an immune system cancer that has to be triggered from some outside source. I will perhaps never know "why me" or how it invaded my body. I will no doubt go to my grave, hopefully as a very old woman, still wondering how that tumor grew inside me and why.

part was not knowing each day how I'd feel when I woke up. But one thing was for sure: I was always tired, but thankful to be alive. A few more months and my grapefruit sized tumor would have been the size of a cantaloupe. It could have killed me then. Thank goodness I pressed my doctor to keep searching.

I was fortunate to have the support of my station and I came up with the idea to put each and every step of my treatment on television on the nightly news each Wednesday evening at 10:00 p.m. We called it "Cherokee's Journal, lessons in living with cancer." People in this state embraced me with open arms because so many of them were going through it with me. Many I heard from didn't make it, many did.

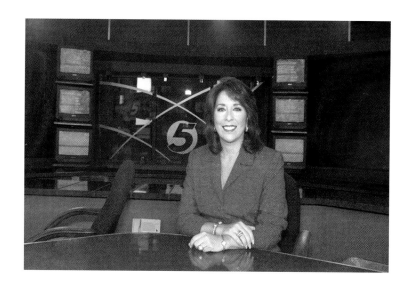

Our thanks to the following places for letting us use
their facilities and services:

Ice Challet, San Mateo, California
The Kohl Mansion, Burlingame, California
Wilshire Garden Market, Oklahoma City, Oklahoma
Channel 5 TV KOCO, Oklahoma City, Oklahoma
The Pin Cushion Fabric Store in Guthrie, Oklahoma
The Guthrie Gun Fighters, Inc., Guthrie, Oklahoma
Fisherman's Warf, Half Moon Bay, California
Espaço Renascer at the Cancer Hospital in Recife, Brazil

Should you wish to contact the photographer or any of the ladies featured in this book, please do so by sending an e-mail to:

icanstilldance@datavisuals.net

Your message will be forwarded to the person you write to.

bloopers...

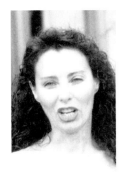

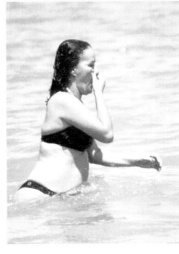

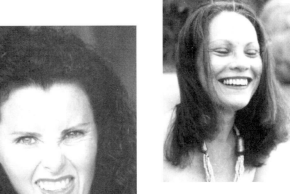

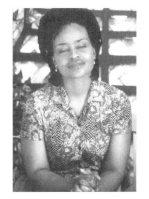

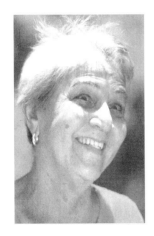

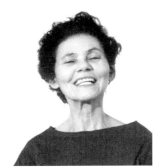

I wasn't ready!...

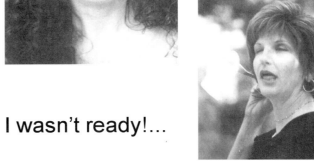

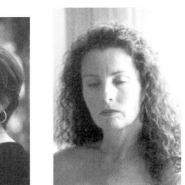

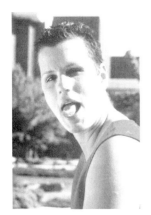

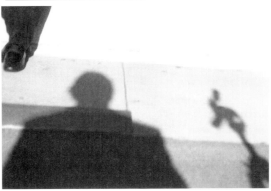

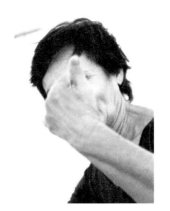

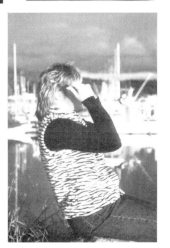

sometimes it's the photographer's fault

... we are beautiful, not perfect!

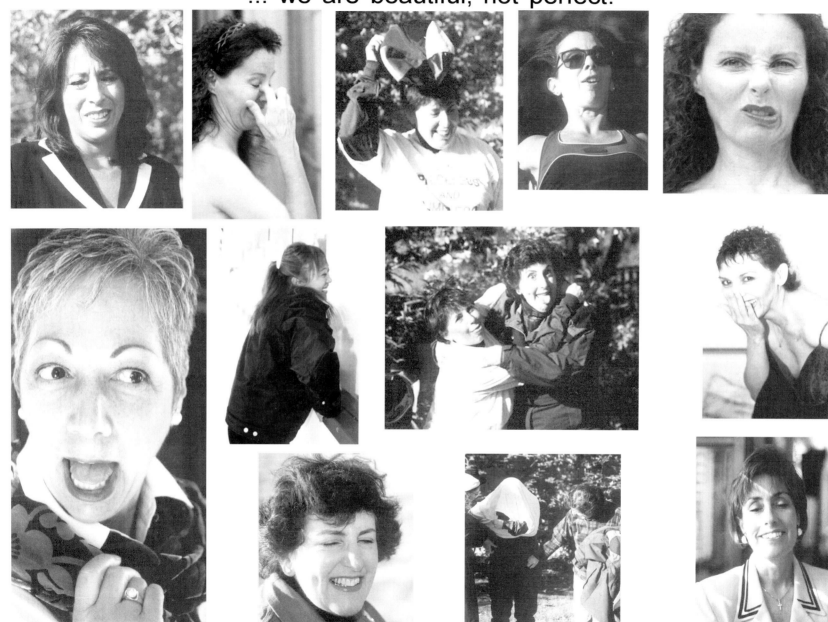

Dictionary

(from the web site of the National Cancer Institute)

adjuvant therapy (AD-joo-vant): Treatment given after the primary treatment to increase the chances of a cure. Adjuvant therapy may include chemotherapy, radiation therapy, or hormone therapy.

areola (a-REE-o-la): The area of dark-colored skin on the breast that surrounds the nipple.

aspirate (AS-pi-rit): Fluid withdrawn from a lump, often a cyst, or a nipple.

atypical hyperplasia (hy-per-PLAY-zha): A benign (noncancerous) condition in which cells have abnormal features and are increased in number.

autologous bone marrow transplantation (aw-TAHL-o-gus): A procedure in which bone marrow is removed from a person, stored, and then given back to the person after intensive treatment.

axilla (ak-SIL-a): The underarm or armpit.

axillary (AK-sil-air-ee): Pertaining to the armpit area, including the lymph nodes that are located there.

axillary lymph node dissection: Surgery to remove lymph nodes found in the armpit region.

benign (beh-NINE): Not cancerous; does not invade nearby tissue or spread to other parts of the body.

biological therapy (by-o-LAHJ-i-kul): Treatment to stimulate or restore the ability of the immune system to fight infection and disease. Also used to lessen side effects that may be caused by some cancer treatments. Also known as immunotherapy, biotherapy, or biological response modifier (BRM) therapy.

biopsy (BY-ahp-see): The removal of cells or tissues for examination under a microscope. When only a sample of tissue is removed, the procedure is called an incisional biopsy or core biopsy. When an entire tumor or lesion is removed, the procedure is called an excisional biopsy. When a sample of tissue or fluid is removed with a needle, the procedure is called a needle biopsy or fine-needle aspiration.

bone marrow: The soft, sponge-like tissue in the center of bones that produces white blood cells, red blood cells, and platelets.

breast reconstruction: Surgery to rebuild a breast's shape after a mastectomy.

breast-conserving surgery: An operation to remove the breast cancer but not the breast itself. Types of breast-conserving surgery include lumpectomy (removal of the lump), quadrantectomy (removal of one quarter of the breast), and segmental mastectomy (removal of the cancer as well as some of the breast tissue around the tumor and the lining over the chest muscles below the tumor).

cancer: A term for diseases in which abnormal cells divide without control. Cancer cells can invade nearby tissues and can spread through the bloodstream and lymphatic system to other parts of the body.

carcinoma (kar-sin-O-ma): Cancer that begins in the skin or in tissues that line or cover internal organs.

chemotherapy (kee-mo-THER-a-pee): Treatment with anticancer drugs.

clinical trial: A research study that tests how well new medical treatments or other interventions work in people. Each study is designed to test new methods of screening, prevention, diagnosis, or treatment of a disease.

colony-stimulating factors: Substances that stimulate the production of blood cells. Colony-stimulating factors include granulocyte colony-stimulating factors (also called G-CSF and filgrastim), granulocyte-macrophage colony-stimulating factors (also called GM-CSF and sargramostim), and promegapoietin.

cyst (sist): A sac or capsule filled with fluid.

duct (dukt): A tube through which body fluids pass.

ductal carcinoma in situ (DUK-tal kar-sin-O-ma in SYE-too): DCIS. Abnormal cells that involve only the lining of a duct. The cells have not spread outside the duct to other tissues in the breast. Also called intraductal carcinoma.

estrogens (ES-tro-jins): A family of hormones that promote the development and maintenance of female sex characteristics.

fine-needle aspiration: The removal of tissue or fluid with a needle for examination under a microscope. Also called needle biopsy.

gene: The functional and physical unit of heredity passed from parent to offspring. Genes are pieces of DNA, and most genes contain the information for making a specific protein.

hormonal therapy: Treatment of cancer by removing, blocking, or adding hormones. Also called hormone therapy or endocrine therapy.

hormone receptor test: A test to measure the amount of certain proteins, called hormone receptors, in cancer tissue. Hormones can attach to these proteins. A high level of hormone receptors may mean that hormones help the cancer grow.

hormone replacement therapy: HRT. Hormones (estrogen, progesterone, or both) given to postmenopausal women or women who have had their ovaries surgically removed, to replace the estrogen no longer produced by the ovaries.

hormones: Chemicals produced by glands in the body and circulated in the bloodstream. Hormones control the actions of certain cells or organs.

hysterectomy (hiss-ter-EK-toe-mee): An operation in which the uterus is removed.

incision (in-SIH-zhun): A cut made in the body during surgery.

infertility: The inability to produce children.

inflammatory breast cancer: A type of breast cancer in which the breast looks red and swollen and feels warm. The skin of the breast may also show the pitted appearance called peau d'orange (like the skin of an orange). The redness and warmth occur because the cancer cells block the lymph vessels in the skin.

invasive cancer: Cancer that has spread beyond the layer of tissue in which it developed and is growing into surrounding, healthy tissues. Also called infiltrating cancer.

lobe: A portion of an organ such as the liver, lung, breast, or brain.

lobular carcinoma in situ (LOB-yoo-lar kar-sin-O-ma in SYE-too): LCIS. Abnormal cells found in the lobules of the breast. This condition seldom becomes invasive cancer; however, having lobular carcinoma in situ increases one's risk of developing breast cancer in either breast.

lobule (LOB-yule): A small lobe or subdivision of a lobe.

local therapy: Treatment that affects cells in the tumor and the area close to it.

lumpectomy (lump-EK-toe-mee): Surgery to remove the tumor and a small amount of normal tissue around it.

lymph (limf): The almost colorless fluid that travels through the lymphatic system and carries cells that help fight infection and disease.

lymph node: A rounded mass of lymphatic tissue that is surrounded by a capsule of connective tissue. Also known as a lymph gland. Lymph nodes are spread out along lymphatic vessels and contain many lymphocytes, which filter the lymphatic fluid (lymph).

lymphatic system (lim-FAT-ik): The tissues and organs that produce, store, and carry white blood cells that fight infection and other diseases. This system includes the bone marrow, spleen, thymus, lymph nodes and a network of thin tubes that carry lymph and white blood cells. These tubes branch, like blood vessels, into all the tissues of the body.

lymphedema (LIMF-eh-DEE-ma): A condition in which excess fluid collects in tissue and causes swelling. It may occur in the arm or leg after lymph vessels or lymph nodes in the underarm or groin are removed or treated with radiation.

magnetic resonance imaging (mag-NET-ik REZ-o-nans IM-a-jing): MRI. A procedure in which a magnet linked to a computer is used to create detailed pictures of areas inside the body.

malignant (ma-LIG-nant): Cancerous; a growth with a tendency to invade and destroy nearby tissue and spread to other parts of the body.

mammogram (MAM-o-gram): An x-ray of the breast.

mammography (mam-OG-ra-fee): The use of x-rays to create a picture of the breast.

mastectomy (mas-TEK-toe-mee): Surgery to remove the breast (or as much of the breast tissue as possible).

medical oncologist (on-KOL-o-jist): A doctor who specializes in diagnosing and treating cancer using chemotherapy, hormonal therapy, and biological therapy. A medical oncologist often serves as the main caretaker of someone who has cancer and coordinates treatment provided by other specialists.

menopause (MEN-o-pawz): The time of life when a woman's menstrual periods stop permanently. Also called "change of life."

menstrual cycle (MEN-stroo-al): The monthly cycle of hormonal changes from the beginning of one menstrual period to the beginning of the next.

menstruation: Periodic discharge of blood and tissue from the uterus. Until menopause, menstruation occurs approximately every 28 days when a woman is not pregnant.

metastasis (meh-TAS-ta-sis): The spread of cancer from one part of the body to another. Tumors formed from cells that have spread are called "secondary tumors" and contain cells that are like those in the original (primary) tumor. The plural is metastases.

microcalcifications (MY-krow-kal-si-fi-KAY-shunz): Tiny deposits of calcium in the breast that cannot be felt but can be detected on a mammogram. A cluster of these very small specks of calcium may indicate that cancer is present.

modified radical mastectomy (mas-TEK-toe-mee): Surgery for breast cancer in which the breast, some of the lymph nodes under the arm, the lining over the chest muscles, and sometimes part of the chest wall muscles are removed.

monoclonal antibodies (MAH-no-KLO-nul AN-tih-BAH-deez): Laboratory-produced substances that can locate and bind to cancer cells wherever they are in the body. Many monoclonal antibodies are used in cancer detection or therapy; each one recognizes a different protein on certain cancer cells. Monoclonal antibodies can be used alone, or they can be used to deliver drugs, toxins, or radioactive material directly to a tumor.

neoadjuvant therapy: Treatment given before the primary treatment. Neoadjuvant therapy can be chemotherapy, radiation therapy, or hormone therapy.

nipple discharge: Fluid coming from the nipple.

ovaries (O-va-reez): The pair of female reproductive glands in which the ova, or eggs, are formed. The ovaries are located in the pelvis, one on each side of the uterus.

pathologist (pa-THOL-o-jist): A doctor who identifies diseases by studying cells and tissues under a microscope.

peripheral stem cell transplantation (per-IF-er-al): A method of replacing blood-forming cells destroyed by cancer treatment. Immature blood cells (stem cells) in the circulating blood that are similar to those in the bone marrow are given after treatment to help the bone marrow recover and continue producing healthy blood cells. Transplantation may be autologous (an individual's own blood cells saved earlier), allogeneic (blood cells donated by someone else), or syngeneic (blood cells donated by an identical twin). Also called peripheral stem cell support.

plastic surgeon: A surgeon who specializes in reducing scarring or disfigurement that may occur as a result of accidents, birth defects, or treatment for diseases.

positron emission tomography scan: PET scan. A computerized image of the metabolic activity of body tissues used to determine the presence of disease.

progesterone (pro-JES-ter-own): A female hormone.

prosthesis (pros-THEE-sis): An artificial replacement of a part of the body.

radiation oncologist (ray-dee-AY-shun on-KOL-o-jist): A doctor who specializes in using radiation to treat cancer.

radiation therapy (ray-dee-AY-shun): The use of high-energy radiation from x-rays, gamma rays, neutrons, and other sources to kill cancer cells and shrink tumors. Radiation may come from a machine outside the body (external-beam radiation therapy), or it may come from radioactive material placed in the body in the area near cancer cells (internal radiation therapy, implant radiation, or brachytherapy). Systemic radiation therapy uses a radioactive substance, such as a radiolabeled monoclonal antibody, that circulates throughout the body. Also called radiotherapy.

radical mastectomy (RAD-ih-kal mas-TEK-toe-mee): Surgery for breast cancer in which the breast, chest muscles, and all of the lymph nodes under the arm are removed. For many years, this was the operation most used, but it is used now only when the tumor has spread to the chest muscles. Also called the Halsted radical mastectomy.

risk factor: A habit, trait, condition, or genetic alteration that increases a person's chance of developing a disease.

screening: Checking for disease when there are no symptoms.

segmental mastectomy (mas-TEK-toe-mee): The removal of the cancer as well as some of the breast tissue around the tumor and the lining over the chest muscles below the tumor. Usually some of the lymph nodes under the arm are also taken out. Sometimes called partial mastectomy.

sentinel lymph node biopsy: Procedure in which a dye or radioactive substance is injected near the tumor and flows into the sentinel lymph nodes(s) (the first lymph node(s) that cancer is likely to spread to from the primary tumor). A surgeon then looks for the dye or uses a scanner to find the sentinel lymph node(s) and removes it (or them) to check for the presence of tumor cells.

stage: The extent of a cancer, especially whether the disease has spread from the original site to other parts of the body.

surgery: A procedure to remove or repair a part of the body or to find out whether disease is present.

systemic (sis-TEM-ik): Affecting the entire body.

tissue (TISH-oo): A group or layer of cells that are alike in type and work together to perform a specific function.

total mastectomy (mas-TEK-toe-mee): Removal of the breast. Also called simple mastectomy.

tumor (TOO-mer): An abnormal mass of tissue that results from excessive cell division. Tumors perform no useful body function. They may be benign (not cancerous) or malignant (cancerous).

ultrasonography (UL-tra-son-OG-ra-fee): A procedure in which sound waves (called ultrasound) are bounced off tissues and the echoes are converted to a picture (sonogram).

x-ray: High-energy radiation used in low doses to diagnose diseases and in high doses to treat cancer.

....

Resources

Your own doctors, nurses or health care providers are your first sources for answers to your questions.

The National Institutes of Health and **The National Cancer Institute's Cancer Information Service** (CSI) publish several booklets containing information about breast cancer diagnosis and treatment.

Telephone: 1-800-4-CANCER (1-800-442-6237)
TTY: 1-800-332-8615
web sites: http://www.nci.nih.gov
                 http://rex.nci.nih.gov
                 http://cancernet.nci.nih.gov
                 http://cancertrials.nci.nih.gov

The Community Breast Health Project in Palo Alto, California, was a fantastic place for me to get the information and some of the help I needed.
web site: www.cbhp.org

Dr. Susan Love's Breast Book was very informative and answered a lot of my questions about breast surgeries and other breast cancer related issues.